THE SCAVENGERS' MANIFESTO

THE
SCAVENGERS'
MANIFESTO

Anneli Rufus
and
Kristan Lawson

JEREMY P. TARCHER/PENGUIN
a member of Penguin Group (USA) Inc.
New York

JEREMY P. TARCHER/PENGUIN
Published by the Penguin Group
Penguin Group (USA) Inc., 375 Hudson Street, New York, New York 10014, USA *
Penguin Group (Canada), 90 Eglinton Avenue East, Suite 700, Toronto, Ontario
M4P 2Y3, Canada (a division of Pearson Canada Inc.) * Penguin Books Ltd, 80 Strand,
London WC2R 0RL, England * Penguin Ireland, 25 St Stephen's Green, Dublin 2, Ireland
(a division of Penguin Books Ltd) * Penguin Group (Australia), 250 Camberwell Road,
Camberwell, Victoria 3124, Australia * (a division of Pearson Australia Group Pty Ltd) *
Penguin Books India Pvt Ltd, 11 Community Centre, Panchsheel Park,
New Delhi–110 017, India * Penguin Group (NZ), 67 Apollo Drive, Rosedale,
North Shore 0632, New Zealand (a division of Pearson New Zealand Ltd) *
Penguin Books (South Africa) (Pty) Ltd, 24 Sturdee Avenue,
Rosebank, Johannesburg 2196, South Africa

Penguin Books Ltd, Registered Offices: 80 Strand, London WC2R 0RL, England

Most Tarcher/Penguin books are available at special quantity discounts for bulk
purchase for sales promotions, premiums, fund-raising, and educational needs.
Special books or book excerpts also can be created to fit specific needs.
For details, write Penguin Group (USA) Inc. Special Markets,
375 Hudson Street, New York, NY 10014.

LIBRARY OF CONGRESS CATALOGING-IN-PUBLICATION DATA
Rufus, Anneli S.
The scavengers' manifesto / Anneli Rufus and Kristan Lawson.
p.   cm.
Includes bibliographical references and index.
ISBN 978-1-58542-717-8
1. Ragpickers—United States.   2. Salvage (Waste, etc.)—United States.
I. Lawson, Kristan.   II. Title.
HD9975.U52R84   2009   2008054636
640—dc22

Printed in the United States of America
1   3   5   7   9   10   8   6   4   2

This book is printed on recycled paper.

Book design by Lovedog Studio

While the authors have made every effort to provide accurate telephone numbers and Internet
addresses at the time of publication, neither the publisher nor the authors assume any
responsibility for errors, or for changes that occur after publication. Further, the publisher does
not have any control over and does not assume any responsibility for author or third-party
websites or their content.

CONTENTS

INTRODUCTION

After this I went every Day on Board, and brought away what I could get. I had been now thirteen Days on Shore, and had been eleven Times on Board the Ship; in which Time I had brought away all that one Pair of Hands could well be suppos'd capable to bring, tho' I believe verily, had the calm Weather held, I should have brought away the whole Ship Piece by Piece: But preparing the 12th Time to go on Board, I found the Wind begin to rise; however at low Water I went on Board, and tho' I thought I had rumag'd the Cabbin so effectually, as that nothing more could be found, yet I discover'd a Locker with Drawers in it, in one of which I found two or three Razors, and one Pair of large Sizzers, with some ten or a Dozen of good Knives and Forks; in another I found about Thirty six Pounds value in Money, some European Coin, some Brazil, some Pieces of Eight, some Gold, some Silver. I smil'd to my self at the Sight.

—DANIEL DEFOE, *Robinson Crusoe*

ALL AROUND THE WORLD, A CHANGE IS NOW AFOOT. The way in which human beings acquire stuff is shifting. Expanding. Forever. All around the world, millions are salvaging stuff, trading stuff, recycling stuff. This is the end of the shopping monopoly.

All around the world, we are scavenging. Today that doesn't mean only the squalid ragpicking it used to mean. So many pursuits count as scavenging today that they can no longer be tucked into any easy little category. We, the authors of this book, redefine scavenging as any way of legally acquiring stuff that does not involve paying full price. Just think how many ways you do this on a daily basis. You scavenge just by tracking down a good bargain.

It used to be that when anyone wanted anything, she automatically rushed out to the store and bought it new, full price. Mission accomplished. Back then—not so long ago—it was assumed that buying things new, retail, was the only way in which respectable civilized human beings could get them. Getting goods by any other means besides store-bought, new, and full price was considered suspicious: fit only for bottom-feeders, moochers, cheapskates, bums.

Four thousand years of prejudice dies hard.

Not long ago, *just a few years ago*, in our corporate consumer culture, the very idea of getting stuff by any means outside the standard retail channel at any speed but warp speed was anathema.

A sacrilege.

A sin.

Not long ago, all of American society pledged loyalty to new-and-improved products. Not-shopping was treason.

An abomination.

In that unquestioning, unevolved age, not so long ago, not-shopping—at least, not shopping new, full price—would have made friends and neighbors call you radical. Antiestablishment. Heck, un-American.

And/or those friends and neighbors would have assumed you

were poor. They might have pitied you. *She must be destitute. Why else wouldn't she like the mall?*

BUT TIMES have changed. A confluence of factors—style, politics, technology, ecology, and the economy—have made more and more of us seek more and more alternate means of acquiring stuff. Modern-day scavengers are bold, committed, and resourceful. Goods and services now circle and recircle the world, connecting strangers, not a penny spent.

The more accepted scavenging becomes, the more of us there are.

And the lesser the prejudices.

Well, that took long enough.

Damned in the Book of Genesis, declared untouchable in the Book of Leviticus, shunned by cultures around the world, we're scavengers.

We're trash-pickers. We're treasure-hunters. Bargain shoppers. Beachcombers. Recyclers. Freecyclers. Sample-sifters. Coupon shoppers. Swappers. Wherever we are, wherever we go, we find ways to not shop.

We don't steal.

We don't scam.

But we don't pay full price. We don't pay at all if we can help it. In which case, to be true to our ethics, the authors feel like saying: *Pssst.* Scavenge this book. Find it in the street. Buy it for spare change at a yard sale or a flea market or a thrift shop. Snatch it from a FREE box. Fish it from a Dumpster—although we hope it would never end up there. Borrow it from the library.

Whoops, there goes our future income.

We seldom know what we will acquire, or where or when or how or even if. But admit it: you love a mystery.

AN E-MAIL that circulated around New York City in May 2008 exhorted:

"Come attend the first planning meeting for the Freegan Fashion Show fundraiser coming up on June 6. The Freegan Fashion Show kicks off with a week of freegan clothing making workshops using scrap material we redeem from the fabric district. Fashion week ends with our models walking the runway and showing how creativity is beautiful and sexy. Create your own style instead of buying a corporate version of your self-identity. This is a big event and all help is appreciated."

TWO THOUSAND years ago, half the world's population still survived by hunting and gathering. Over the last four hundred years, traditional hunting and gathering has, in the strictest sense, become nearly extinct. But *all* modern-day scavengers—whether at thrift shops or in Dumpsters or in CurbCycle groups or at yard sales—are in some sense hunter-gatherers. Define hunting-gathering as foraging, taking what comes. Define it as sublimating *choice* to the bigger thrill of *chance*. It translates to saving money and potentially working less. It translates to dodging whatever market sector some genius thinks you belong to. Modern scavenging means wearing discards cast off by a throng of strangers, thus you can't be deciphered. *You* are the mystery. Hunting and gathering downtown, eyes to the ground in an urban landscape, the authors of this book found, in one week: a pearl-and-amber earring, four free-sample cans of pomegranate soda, two empty wire-handled five-gallon plastic vats, three bus transfers worth twenty-five cents apiece, a mysterious doohickey that turned out to be a digital pedometer, eighty-seven cents in change, and a ten-dollar bill. One day we plucked a clutch of perfumey, fuzzy-fleshed, creamy-meated Chinese loquats from a dark-leafed tree. Some days we find nothing. Last Saturday we bought an electric hedge trimmer at a yard sale for two bucks. Later that day, in a box marked FREE, we found fourteen shirts. We go days at a span without even opening our wallets. Our garden grows with scavenged seeds. Sometimes we do not know what they are when we plant them and find out only when plants come up: tomatoes, collards, tomatillos, parsley, three kinds of bok choy. You never know.

That is the point.

That is the challenge and the payoff and the thrill of scavenging: the never knowing, then the accidental reward. *And can you handle the unknown?*

In a paved-over world, the modern scavenger reclaims discovery.

The modern scavenger reclaims the quest.

We, the authors of this book, have scavenged for as long as we can remember. We didn't know each other when we were kids—lived in different cities far apart, though contemporaneously. Yet each of us, in his or her own way, was foraging, scrounging, saving, and repurposing practically as soon as he or she could walk and talk. One of us lived near a beach and was frequently taken there. Found shells, smooth pebbles, sea glass, driftwood, sand, and dried seaweed turned into countless dollhouse furnishings and early art projects even before the first day of first grade. Another of us lived in a town studded with hippie communes, whose residents demonstrated how to construct furniture from scrap wood and to pick plums from sidewalk trees. One of us was mocked by classmates for picking up spare change from the street or sidewalk. The other one searched for coins at the feet of parking meters first thing in the morning in order to buy lunch at school. Ten years before we met, both of us bought metal detectors, in both cases the cheapest Radio Shack model. One of us trolled the beach. The other trolled parks and playgrounds. In college, still not having yet met, we filled our closets with thrift-shop clothes, our shelves with secondhand textbooks, and our fridges with leftovers from the restaurants where we worked. Once we met, neither of us ever had to explain or apologize to the other for bending down to pick up coins or standing on tiptoes to peer inside Dumpsters. In all these years, choosing the least expensive item, place, or option has never sparked a spat. We do not socialize with others much, for better or worse. We know that, behind our backs, others surmise that we are parsimonious or poor. Or they remember encounters like this: One day we were at the home of a friend when she realized that she needed to jot a quick note for the postal carrier. A trash bag at her feet was full of scrap paper on which she could have jotted it: torn envelopes, wrappers, receipts. Rather than grab one of these and scribble the note on it, she sighed, strode over to a desk, opened a drawer, and pulled a sheet of thick, expensive stationery from a silver box. Upon this creamy monogrammed sheet, she scribbled: "Leave packages on porch." "Okay," she said, and stood.

We gazed at her as if she were an alien.

She gazed back at us the same way.

We blanched at her brash, mindless, needless waste. *A perfectly good sheet of blank paper.*

And she thought: *What?*

Sometimes scavenging is the Great Divide.

———

WE BRING plastic bags everywhere we go, folded small, tucked into pockets, because we never know what we might find. They're especially handy for fruit gleaned from the innumerable sidewalk trees in our neighborhood. We *do* know: Free is the best price.

Not all scavengers scavenge with the same goals in mind. Yes, we want free stuff—or at least cheap stuff. From that point on, we diverge.

Fine.

SOME SCAVENGE for fun. Some scavenge to save. Money. The world. While millions all around us drown in debt, we liberate ourselves with every cent we save while liberating tons of would-be garbage. We know that the difference between brand-new, full-price products and their scratched secondhand counterparts is—

Debt.

Some scavenge to recycle. Repurpose. Reduce. Reuse. They know that some 254 million tons of trash is thrown out every year in the United States alone. In New York City, 64,000 tons *per week*.

Some scavenge to revolt.

Some scavenge to survive.

Some scavenge for the sake of spontaneity. The long-forgotten magic of the random.

Some scavenge for art. Some scavenge for adventure. Some scavenge for self-sufficiency. For some, scavenging is a test. For some, it's spiritual.

We do not all scavenge for the same reasons, yet we share

certain understandings, certain values, certain principles. We share a way of life. A way of looking at the world. Having, each of us, shattered the chains that locked us to consumer culture, we walk free under a clear new sky, scanning a changed terrain studded with buried treasure.

This book is our manifesto and our map.

We seek but do not always find. This makes each find a miracle.

Amen.

CONSUMER CULTURE causes atrophy. Instant gratification renders the gratified lazy. Weak. Incurious. Consumers say they would never be scavengers because—they say—they could not stand the sacrifice. They say, *I deserve better*. They say, *I deserve the best*. They say, *I love myself too much to collect junk*.

We will not let ourselves be told what is worth what.

THIS MIGHT BE the last book you ever buy.

CHAPTER 1

FREE YOUR MIND

The Philosophy of
Scavenging

ON A HOT SUMMER SATURDAY, WE ARE RUSHING—
late—to a family birthday party. We are rushing; we've told
each other: Not one more delay. But then we see a yard-
sale sign.

And wordlessly we diverge from our route, follow the
arrow on the sign and arc left to where we see balloons and
clamor halfway down the block, and *ahhh*.

It's not just any yard sale but a big one, stretching from the
sidewalk, where blue satin cushions lean against a stop sign,
up a driveway studded with chairs, and across a front lawn
strewn with clothes, books, tools, kitchenware, toys. As luck
would have it, this yard sale is ending just as we arrive. From
her porch, the seller announces that the sale is over and that
everything remaining is now free for the taking.

Not all sales end this way. Some sellers pack their unsold
stuff back up and haul it inside or drive it to Goodwill. Some,

though, give it all away. When word gets out, a buzz goes through the air and everything speeds up. Hands dart. Receptacles are sought to hold the DVDs, the baseball mitt, the vase.

This is a free-for-all.

At any free-for-all, you can immediately spot the inexperienced. Gobsmacked, they hover over pomanders and clocks but reach for nothing, as if fearing germs or tricks or that they will be called thieves.

And you can spot the scavengers. We glide, our movements purposeful and lithe. Our eyes cut wide arcs, back and forth. We gaze from side to side, like lighthouse beacons, even as we kneel and reach with one hand for shirts—*stripes, button-down, yes*—and with the other for swim goggles, garden gloves, a blender. Yoink! Into the backpack pops the spoon, the copper horse, the coffeepot. Quick. Competent. Assess each item in a nanosecond. Do I want this? Do I need it? Show it to a friend and ask: Do you?

We will be late to the family party. And when we get there and they ask why we are late and we say we were scavenging free clothes and toys and kitchenware from a stranger's front lawn, they laugh. When they see we are serious, they withdraw from us with shocked looks and ask: But why? Wasn't it dirty? What if someone bled on those shirts? What if someone cooked meth in that coffeepot? What if the blender's broken? Can't you afford new goggles?

Oh, *that*. We hear it all the time.

And more:

What if it doesn't fit?

What if it's dented/scratched/stained/faded/ripped?

Wouldn't you rather just go to a store and buy the exact color/size/style/components that you like best?

What are you going to do with that?

Do you even know what it is?

DON'T LET ME BE MISUNDERSTOOD

Admit that you have scavenged anything and you can automatically expect questions. Misconceptions. Misperceptions. Even accusations. Thousands of years of prejudice die hard. Most non-scavengers—we call them *standard consumers*—recoil at the very thought of *not* buying things brand-new at full price. They never question this. Standard consumers presume that theirs is the *only* way to acquire, that any other way reeks of squalor or theft.

How do we tell them how it is for us? How do we tell them that, for us, old stuff and stuff that has been owned before acquires a patina composed of history and mystery, almost a soul? How do we say that a shiny new nickel is just cash to us but an oxidized greenish 1954 nickel, worn so smooth that Thomas Jefferson lacks eyes, excites us, sets our minds skittering up and down the years, wondering, *Who held this coin, where, when, why?* How do we tell standard consumers that new merchandise bores and depresses us? That mass production makes *them* into drones? How do we tell them we despair for those who spend sixty-five dollars at the store on the same shirt that costs (or will, within a year) three dollars at the thrift shop? How can we explain the size of landfills, the amount of solid waste now littering the Earth? Do we cite findings by the Clean Air Council that every American alive discards fifty-six tons of trash per year? Do we mention the millions of pounds of trash floating on the seas? Do we say that, by scavenging, we can make a dent in these figures?

How do we tell them we appreciate our scavenged goods in ways they cannot possibly appreciate their brand-new full-price purchases? How can we say that every scavenged item came to us in a unique, often unexpected way, so each one adds another story to our lives? How can we say: Full-price shopping is easy, but scavenging takes talent, luck, skill, and expertise? Thus every scavenged item is a reward or a miracle. How can we explain that not paying full price for things gives us the best assessment of true value: we appreciate our scavenged goods not for how much they cost us but for what they have been through and what they are.

How can we tell standard consumers that every saved penny counts, that saved pennies add up? They call us cheap. They call us poor. Yet the average standard consumer carries a four-figure debt. How can we make them understand that they accumulated these debts by paying full price? How can we say: What would you prefer—discount-outlet food, library DVDs to watch, and no debt; or restaurant food, cinema tickets, and debt? How do we show them that what they would call insufferable sacrifices set us free?

Do we say: We shrink landfills?

Do we say: We are archaeologists?

Do we say: Not buying at full price makes us creative, independent, self-sufficient, clear-sighted, communitarian, appreciative, liberated, and adventurous?

Do we say: Finding stuff is fun?

Do we say: Money saved is *money saved*?

Wait. We just did.

FINDING AS IDENTITY

We always find stuff. We two authors. Us.

We find stuff everywhere: some of it you would want, some you would not. The Ray-Ban sunglasses. Ripe apricots. The life-sized lifelike rubber vampire bat, with rubber string for easy, bouncy hanging. None of it our choice, but that's the point. We find it, but more likely it finds us. Sometimes we feel like it's almost cosmic, like we're plugged into some kind of magic network, like we find certain stuff at certain times for certain reasons. *Shhh,* though. That's too weird. Don't tell.

We pluck nickels from gutters, toasters from thrift-shop shelves, and Kate Spade bags from other people's trash. When one of us was six, her father asked what she would be when she grew up. She said she didn't know. A nurse, her father said, a ballerina? She said no. He snorted: Okay then—a beachcomber? He was trying to be sarcastic. She took it as instructions. *Okay, Dad!* Imagining the palm-frond hat, the shack.

It has come true.

Scavenging, finding the slightly damaged radio, the box of wartime-Tokyo photographs, feels like rescue, feels like recovery, feels like discovery.

It feels like victory.

Some scavenged finds feel like gifts whose meaning—hmmm, a deck of transparent playing cards—we will someday grasp. This makes them numinous. If we have any faith, it is in luck. Everyday grails. Some scavengers procure commodities: they barter and re-sell. For some, scavenging is an ethos, not a source of income but an income extender, just as Hamburger Helper extends ground beef. The more we find, the less we buy.

Some, like us, can't bring ourselves to eat food rescued from Dumpsters; others don't flinch. We all have our limits. But still:

We, the authors, have not bought new clothes in twelve years. We last bought an umbrella in 1996. Faced with a choice, we always ask: Is there a way to do this, get this, eat this legally for free? It is a reflex. *Not* scavenging feels unnatural. Just going somewhere, paying full price for something, as everyone else does, feels weird.

We live in the land of the (literally) free.

To us, ten dollars is a lot. Hell, *three* dollars is a lot.

Scavengers touch the ground: Not clean, you say. Bacterial spumoni, you say. Who dares finger the sidewalk and street? The scavenger as vector. In actual fact, the ground is not so bad. We ride buses and trains and watch what respectable-looking people smear on rails and straps and seats. *That's* gross. And yet dignified commuters blithely join this viral potluck every day. Nonetheless, scavengers disgust you.

Scavengers are the last still-scornable scapegoats in an almost open-minded world.

Just as each of us has our limits, each scavenger nurses his or her own secret dream of the ultimate find: the treasure-trove-*pour-moi* whose value might be monetary but might not, the elusive not-yet-found find that will be an epiphany. No two such dreams are quite alike, these El Dorados not of longitude and latitude but of that fragile equation: right time, right place. That we could simply buy these items is irrelevant. *They must be found.* We know a man still awaiting a sextant.

MANY TYPES OF SCAVENGER, ONE SHARED MIND-SET

These days, more activities count as scavenging than you might imagine. To us, scavenging means any way in which goods can be acquired for less than full price. This could mean thrift shops. Flea markets. Metal detecting. Freecycling. Coupon clipping. Plain old sales. All of these and more are forms of scavenging. And all remove us from that soulless, processed, debt-provoking standard retail cycle. Finding alternatives, establishing a separate system we call "scavenomics," we inhabit our own world-within-a-world that feels to us like a hunt and like heaven and like home.

We can't be lumped together. You and I and that goateed guy

reaching at the same time for the free books at the yard sale and free brownies at the gallery reception might never be friends. We might fight over sports or politics or style. We might draw blood. We neither look nor talk alike. We don't even scavenge alike. Some of us thrift-shop. Others Dumpster-dive. Some of us hunt treasure. Others trade junk. Some, including both authors of this book, are nonstop wherever-whenever scavengers for whom almost every experience becomes a scavenging experience. Ninety-nine percent of what we now own we got for free.

Some of us use/eat/wear our finds. Others make their finds into crafts, or even fine art. Some scavenge to feed their kids. Some scavenge to save the world.

Yet in a lot of ways, we think and feel alike.

FREAKS

First: We are freaks. Not in our own eyes (hopefully), but in the eyes of most people for most of history. This is improving now, as we shall see, but underscoring any scavenger philosophy must be the fact that what we do is still mainly considered strange and gross and bad. So also underscoring any scavenger philosophy is the fact that we should *have* a philosophy in the first place. That way, we can clarify what makes us scavenge, what sets us apart.

And celebrate ourselves.

No MATTER how or why you do it, even if you're just re-using Christmas ribbon or picking fruit in a vacant lot, you are a radical.

You are acquiring and/or having-without-buying goods that the establishment, the seemingly omnipotent consumer culture in which we were born and raised, insists that we must buy. In refusing to buy—at least, in refusing to pay full price—we are capitalism's naughty children, little rebels, sprinting through the gate.

This culture is conceived, created, operated on the premise that every man, woman, and child should shop as much as possible. The presumption is that this shopping will be standard retail: brand-new, mass-produced, full price. And this presumption permeates every aspect of modern life. We are bred to associate every activity with buying something. Much of modern identity is shaped by what kind of shopper you are. We are bred, in this culture, to define each other by how much we spend and where, on what.

Scavengers step out of this loop. We cannot be read or defined according to the measurements a consumer culture says to use. So in one sense, we are invisible. In one sense, we do not exist.

What does consumer culture see when it sees scavengers?

It sees oddballs who do not spend enough or do not spend at all. *Consumer culture hates this.* It sees oddballs who touch trash. *Consumer culture fears this.* It sees independent oddballs who think for themselves. *Consumer culture fears this most of all.*

By rejecting the standard retail cycle, scavengers reverse the basic order of consumerthink. That is: *want-get.* From infancy, standard consumers learn that whatever they want, they get. They *must* get it. They *will.* Right *now.* Whatever it costs. *Now.* Consumer culture teaches that instant gratification is a basic human right. Consumer culture teaches that waiting is torture. Consumer culture teaches: You are entitled to whatever you desire. *Volo, ergo sum.*

SCAVENGERS SWITCH THAT. Not buying things at full price pretty much mandates having to wait. Depending on your mode of scavenging, it might mean waiting for a sale. It might mean: stop and comparison-shop. It might mean eschewing the closest (most expensive) store and waiting to visit a cheaper one farther away. Scavenging might mean not shopping at ordinary stores. Discount and thrift shopping entails the possibility of not finding what you seek right away. It might be weeks before a red angora short-sleeved sweater turns up at the local Goodwill. And will it be in your size? We wait. Or we *get something else, not what we thought we wanted in the first place.* Chuck that want and get the white lambswool long-sleeved sweater instead.

Then again, scavenging might mean not shopping at stores, period. Who knows when what you think you want will turn up at a flea market or yard sale? Wait, wait, wait. Get something else. Then again, for some of us, scavenging means *not shopping any-where.* It means *not spending anything.* Who knows when what you think you want will turn up in a FREE box, in a trash can, on the ground, or at a swap?

The very principle of scavenging makes want-get pretty much impossible. It also makes want-get seem ludicrous. Especially the way we see want-get enacted all around us: like the screaming-pouting-pounding of spoiled brats.

Scavengers do not expect to get everything we want.

Thus we want less.

We get—whatever comes our way. Wherever and whenever. We are grateful then. But we do not spend our days driven to satisfy our wants.

We can't.

For us it is: *get-want.*

We always get *something,* sooner or later. But in flipping the equation, scavengers have traded choice for chance.

We like chance. Relish chance. Removing standard shopping from our lives means removing a major source of certainty, that is, want-get. It is that certainty on which standard consumers base their lives, which they think is a right, and on which they rely. Removing it from our lives is the only fundamental choice scavengers make.

Scavengers choose to never choose.

And by eschewing certainty and choice—*by choice*—scavengers hold a separate set of values. An exciting, inspiring, invigorating set.

We sing the consumer anthem backward. No wonder we scare society.

DEFERRED CONSUMPTION

Here in the realm of the random, scavengers feel no sense of entitlement.

Immersed in a consumer culture, we do not really consume.

Out here in the realm of the random, scavengers cannot be greedy—because we depend on the lost and discarded, on what others do not want.

For the same reason, we cannot be haughty.

Cannot make demands.

Cannot be ingrates.

Cannot be intolerant.

FOR SCAVENGERS, the world is a roulette wheel. Okay, a roulette wheel whose results we can influence slightly by enhancing certain skills. We relinquish want-get, but our own vigilance and perseverance affects how much or little of whatever we get we get. But basically, in principle: a roulette wheel. So while standard consumers' hearts and minds are consumed by desire, demand, and the impulse to buy, scavengers' hearts and minds have different contours, different impulses.

We wait. We watch. We improvise.

We prefer to defer.

Over time, waiting, watching, improvising, and preferring to defer affect our personalities, we become patient, curious, spontaneous, courageous, flexible, resourceful, optimistic, self-reliant, practical, and easily amused. What comes our way, via FREE box or yard sale or free-sample coupon or trash can? The celadon coffee cup, the Jesus night-light, the white satin sheets, the diamond ring, the power drill, the iPod. Every day brings one more rescue operation, one more foreign expedition, another initiation, one more walk into the wild.

THE DEFINING ACTIVITY in a consumer culture is consumption. To reject the standard *manner* of that activity and do the opposite—in our case, we don't buy—is to make a ferocious statement. A consumer culture is all about getting stuff. But how? *The manner matters.*

In consumer cultures, everything becomes like shopping. The selling of the want-get principle began as a marketing and economic stratagem for selling as much merchandise as possible. To keep a population shopping, supply its every demand while stoking more. Supply those. Stoke again. In mirrors, consumers see want-shaped selves. They have been taught that the more and harder they crave, the more they get, the more alive they are. Consumer culture comprises the constant cultivation and instant gratification of desire. For most consumers, biting into that Big Mac, driving that Eldorado, pulling on that

Baby Phat top feels like mainlining their favorite drug and, to them, feels like victory. Marketers have so mesmerized consumers that consumers see brand logos as *their own logos*, their new flags. Today the brand is the new nation, the new army, the new clan, the new religion, the new tribe. Consumers by the billions line up behind logos, vanish into logos, pour their income into brands.

Yet they discard almost as fast as they consume. And certainly as much. We know they will. Thousands of tons of garbage is collected *each day just in New York City*. The main by-product of want-get is get-waste.

WASTE NOT, WANT NOT

Scavengers *hate* waste.

Of course, we depend on the constant presence of a certain quantity of waste. Discards are our supplies. If all consumers stopped discarding stuff, what could we scavenge? The more waste, the more for us.

Okay. So, in a certain sense, we also *love* waste, since we benefit from it.

But as we rescue other people's waste to repurpose, recycle, and reuse, we hate the principle of waste. We are constantly shocked at what others discard and how much. Better than anyone, we who wade daily through their cast-offs know how warped hearts and minds must be to discard so much. We would rather adopt some bruised, imperfect, thrown-out but still-useful thing than buy a new one because throwing out such stuff seems like a crime to us.

The waste train stops with us.

———

IN FORGOING our "right" to choose, we forgo the privilege to personalize. If our stuff once belonged to others, if *they* chose it first, what makes our stuff feel like it's ours?

Consumers are bred to believe that ever-more-specific versions of mass-produced products are more *theirs*. Not just a cup of house blend but a Grande Mint Mocha Chip Frappuccino Light Blended Coffee with soy milk and two squirts of caramel syrup and four shakes of cinnamon. That's me! Consumers believe the delusion that personal*ized* products are really *personal*. Six hundred cable channels so that you can pick only your favorite shows. *Your* shows. Sixteen iPod colors to choose from, but *my* color is tangerine.

Not orange. Tangerine.

Given a choice, scavengers are as glad as anyone to take our pick. Preferences are natural. But our modes of acquisition pretty much preclude preferences. I like thick-crust pizza best, but if this two-for-one coupon buys only thin-crust, what the heck. I would prefer a plain black watchband to a plaid one, but this practically new Swatch watch I found in the park is plaid. What am I gonna do—discard a perfectly good watch because the band isn't my first choice of color?

Yes, sometimes we will forgo scavenging items that fall *too* far from our taste. Free lipstick in a shade that turns us green? T-shirt bearing a picture of the candidate we hate? We draw the line. But almost always, scavengers cede preference to acceptance. Ninety-nine times out of a hundred, whatever we find, we try. This way, we learn a lot. We broaden our experience. I've never tried yam ice cream before, never worn a poncho, never played this game before, listened to this band, used this device, read this author, seen this film. And *never* would have, had I not scavenged this thing. What we wear/use/eat/do is based on *what we scavenge.* That is: whatever we find for cheap. Whatever we find for free.

Whatever we find.

We cannot cling so tightly to any one motif that it defines, describes, or proscribes us.

We will try anything once. This pries open our minds.

We have walked countless miles in countless others' shoes. And in their coats, their hats, their lost and thrown-out sunscreen.

For scavengers, diversity is not a duty or a novelty but a necessity.

We sublimate what others think is personality to serendipity.

We sacrifice rules to the random.

THIS, TOO, terrifies consumers. They cling desperately to store-bought personality. We prefer not knowing what we will get. *What are you*, consumers would ask us. *Martyrs? Buddhists? Dead?*

And while this trait indeed renders some of us real or inadvertent Buddhists, accidental Taoists, and biblical gleaners-in-the-field, the secular version is this:

We like surprises.

In a processed, paved-over, predictable consumer culture, surprises are rare. That primal, incomparable thrill—*Hello, what's this?*—harks back to an age before brands were flags and stores civilizations. Surprise harks back to a natural, spontaneous world in which anything can happen. Good things. Bad things. In between. But *beyond our control*, and all the more awesome for that.

Whether we scavenge nonstop or selectively, it always entails a surprise. When we eschew want-get, we never know what we will get or where or when or how or even if. This sustains sensations in us that standard consumers lost long ago. Uncertainty. Search-and-discovery. The sudden hallelujah.

Standard consumers are relatively numb to these. A thirst for surprise has been doggedly bred out of them. Consumer culture teaches them: Surprise is dangerous.

Sometimes it is.

Sometimes surprises ache. Sometimes they make your day. They are sunbursts and lightning cracks that make you feel totally real because surprises can't be replicated, can't be duplicated, can't be manufactured, can't be packaged, can't be mass-produced.

You can't predict them. That's the point.

Surprise is absolutely raw.

AND IT IS for the sake of surprise that we are willing to withdraw from mainstream society. For surprise's sake we are willing to depart from expectations, scare and disappoint our families, suffer being tagged bizarre.

IN CHOOSING not to choose, we also get:

Suspense.

We wait to find and we wait to find out.

Standard consumers cannot stand suspense. They try to control time. We know we cannot. Scavenging is open-ended, the results always indefinite. Even the most efficient and active scavenging is slower, with less guaranteed success than a trip to the retail store. Shopping online, for that matter, is instantaneous.

Scavengers live in ambient, nonstop suspense. To us it is a game. A test. A covenant. When it happens it happens, says the scavenger. We wait. We hope. Some pray. And who knows what might happen in the meantime? Suspense always ends with a surprise, for better or worse. This sharpens the senses. It requires faith. We wait and we anticipate.

Patience is multipurpose. The patience we learn by being scavengers is handy in other aspects of life: in crises, most of all. Patience is like a muscle. It is scavengers' gluteus maximus: we use it all day, every day. If we can wait a lifetime for a treasure we may or may not find, *ever*, we can wait for anything.

A FRIEND of ours has always suffered from terrible dental problems. A childhood sweet tooth combined with early-onset lactose intolerance and hippie parents meant not enough calcium, not enough fluoride, lots of cavities, and intermittent dental care at best. Recently he decided enough was enough: he was going to get his teeth fixed at last. He went to a dentist, but got bad news: he needed a permanent bridge to fill a gap where three front teeth were rotting or missing, but first he would need to make as many as ten visits over several months; he needed root canals and caps; he needed teeth pulled; he needed preparatory orthodontics. Only then could the bridge be measured and installed.

After a second visit, he met us for lunch one day, sat down, and flashed a dazzling, enormous smile. "How do you like it?" He beamed. "Pretty amazing, huh?" He then reached into his mouth and—*pop!*—removed a set of realistic plastic front teeth, revealing his familiar yellow stubs underneath. The false teeth resembled fangs from a Halloween costume, but better made and without the sharp incisors. Our friend explained that the dentist had sold him this "temporary bridge" to protect his teeth while the other work was being done. "But," he confided, "I like them so much, I'm just going to use these *instead* of the bridge. I'm never going back!" And with that he popped them back in and handed us a brochure the dentist had given him. "Your teeth aren't so great," our friend said. "You might want to try a set yourself."

We quickly realized that the dentist had given him the wrong brochure. Instead of one intended for the end user, it was a sales brochure that the manufacturer distributes to dentists. And it read: *Many low-income patients requiring long-term dental care abandon the procedures partway through, often leading to further complications. Such patients are now characterized as having Immediate Gratification Syndrome. SmileSaversPro are designed for the IGS sufferer in mind. SmileSaversPro will help you provide at least minimum care for patients not likely to return for the full course of treatment. If you have patients you suspect are suffering from Immediate Gratification Syndrome, contact your supplier for product information.*

(Note: The actual names of the product and the syndrome mentioned above have been changed for privacy's sake.)

What shocked us more than the revelation of a new medical condition called "Immediate Gratification Syndrome" was the uncanny diagnostic accuracy of this new dentist: our friend *did* suffer from a tertiary case of Immediate Gratification Syndrome, but we'd never known that this trait had a name until we read the brochure. Whenever our chain-smoking friend wanted a cigarette, he didn't simply want a cigarette. He wanted one RIGHT. NOW. He was known to pull over on the median strips of freeways to search for a missing pack. Twice he was kicked off airplanes for lighting up while they were taxiing on the runway. Nor was his IGS limited to cigarettes. If he woke up at three a.m. with a craving for blackberry pie, he'd scramble into some clothes, hop into his car, and drive twenty miles to the all-night diner for a slice. His romantic relationships were, as you might imagine, inevitably disastrous. And he was perpetually broke, because money burned holes in his pockets.

But our friend is not alone. Our entire society seems to suffer from Immediate Gratification Syndrome. And the only cure is a healthy dose of scavenging therapy.

SWEET SACRIFICE

Scavengers go without.

We have no beef with wanting stuff. We have no beef with having stuff. Scavengers need not swear off possessions and need not vow to be minimalist antimaterialists. Some are. Some are not. All are scavengers nevertheless. Our beef (well, one of many) is rather with the increasing speed and ease with which consumer culture lets things be acquired, places be reached, and tasks be completed. At first glance, nothing's wrong with speed and ease. Both make the sick and injured safe and well. But speed and ease are habit-forming. They can atrophy body and mind. By making acquisition instantaneous and easy, consumer culture turns populations not just into addicts but addicted insubstantial weaklings. Human marshmallows.

Instantaneity drains everything of meaning. Because scavenging makes acquisition slower, scavenging *slows . . . everything . . . down.* On purpose. Scavengers hear themselves breathe. To savor each morsel, each minute, every day is strangely calming. Yes, we are anachronisms. Yes, we suffer, but our suffering makes the eventual rewards so sweet.

Suffering teaches.

Living with uncertainty requires faith. Not necessarily religious faith, though for some scavengers it is exactly that. But even the most secular among us has faith in the random, faith in chance. Scavengers have faith in patience rewarded. Faith in vigilance and sacrifice repaid. Call it belief in magic. Call it optimism. When we depend not just on what we find but on the process of seek-ing/hunting/waiting/watching/finding, what choice do we have but to believe that we will seek/hunt/wait/watch/find again?

That is: faith in fate *and* faith in ourselves.

Pessimists cannot last long as scavengers.

WHAT DO WE NEED?

Consumer culture blurs the difference between need and want. We are never supposed to know the difference. Standard consum-ers are so pampered that they do not know. Advertisements use both words interchangeably. As a result, standard consumers an-guish all day over phantom needs. They cry, *I NEED a good pinot noir to go with this cheese,* leap into their cars, rush to stores, and buy—while scavengers shrug, stay home, and relax, sipping what-ever already is there.

Do you *need* a eucalyptus-scented plug-in electric air freshener with thirty-day replacement pack, one for each room in the house? No. What you *need* is a tourniquet for that knife wound in your leg. Priorities.

Scavengers know the meaning of need.

We put most so-called needs on hold. Often, we are compelled to employ foresight, looking way ahead. We might decide: *I'll eventually need more bricks to finish this garden wall* and *I need to get Jen and Dave a wedding gift.* At that point, we go on alert for bricks and whatever might constitute a gift. As scavengers, we are always on alert anyway—but once we say *I need,* a special scanning mechanism locks and loads, a long-range, long-term hypervigi-lance, beeping gently away. And when and if we find free bricks (a nearby church tore down its toolshed, say), and when and if the thrift shop gets an antique seder plate, our needs are met. If not, we wait. In a pinch, if time runs out and our needs remain unmet, of course we have to break down and buy retail: Replace that smashed window. Refill this prescription. Then again, we might just build the garden wall not with bricks but with rocks. We might give Jen and Dave that kitschy tiki in our basement. They've always admired it.

HONING THE SENSES

Scavengers see.

We are always watchful, scanning every scene for telltale shapes, colors, and signs that literally or figuratively say: TAKE ME, I'M YOURS. We are the kind who sleep with eyes half open. For us, this is basic math: Look more, find more. Observe, retrieve. Look over, under, sideways, down. Scavengers marvel at how few folks look down while they walk. Most folks stride staring straight ahead, as if to prove themselves progressive and connected. They look down on looking down.

Scavengers strive to see all with our lighthouse-beacon gazes. We filter out nothing, dismiss nothing, no matter how small. Any detail might be a clue. Look here, Watson: what appears to be the sleeve of a pink silk blazer is dangling over the edge of this discarded box. Look here, Watson: behind a storefront window, individuals who do not seem to know each other are staring at sculptures while carrying paper plates. Aha. Art gallery reception, free refreshments, open to the public. Look here, Watson: sinuous white strands tipped with thumbnail-sized white disks are dangling off the curb. Aha. A pair of ear-buds.

Being watchful gains us more than merely stuff. Being watchful means not missing anything. The more we see, the more we know. The more we see, the better entertained. The more we see, the likelier we are to unveil mysteries, espy marvels on the fly. Scavengers are often eavesdroppers as well, scavenging carelessly mishandled secrets of the human heart.

SCAVENGERS IMPROVISE.

No bread? Ran out of wrapping paper? Broken shoelace? Standard consumers rush out to replace lost or broken things with perfect replicas, brand-new, full price. Not scavengers. For us, lost and broken things are hassles but also challenges. We wish our stuff would never disappear or break but every absence or booboo is a brainteaser. We use expired calendar pages instead of wrapping paper. Potatoes instead of bread. Knot the shoelace, of course. Or replace it with ribbon, fishing line.

Improvisation forces us to think. Act. Try.

Experiment.

Like pioneers, we exemplify DIY.

And when it works, we thank ourselves.

An actual example: Some ideas in this chapter came to mind like a bolt from the blue during a solitary walk through an elegant residential neighborhood. No paper or writing utensils had been brought along. Nor were such items anywhere apparent. It was a houses-only district with no businesses of any kind. Nor was anyone visible. Ideas are miracles, scavenged out of thin air. But these risked disappearing if not written down. They were too numerous to memorize. Writing them down could trigger even more. But how? Lacking the means to write felt like being a prehistoric hunter in the wild without a club, slingshot, or stone. Two choices: Prematurely end a lovely walk while straining to remember the ideas, rush home, and write them down. Or stay out there and—

Scavenge.

Pick one: hope or no hope.

Scavenge—or surrender.

The answer was obvious.

The walk became a hunt. For scavengers, all walks are anyway. But now it was a hunt on high alert.

A quest.

The notion of the quest has morphed in the last century. Quests once entailed both the material and the immaterial: Imagine the immensity, in technologically primitive times, of traveling to distant places. Seeing legendary peaks or pilgrimage sites. Circling the world. Speed and ease and the weakness they induce eclipsed the quest.

Paper and writing implement. Paper and writing implement. It formed a background rhythm to the walk, the hunt, the silently chanted ideas. Each mansion on those tree-lined streets was no doubt packed with this absurdly common prey: surely thousands of pens and blank pages rested behind those walls, off-limits. Trash had been collected that day, so the bins along the curbs were empty. Nor was this the sort of district where things are stapled to phone poles. Litter always defines a neighborhood. Near schools: snack wrappers, fast-food wrappers, barrettes, pens and paper. But a wealthy neighborhood like this: litter-free, a scavenger's nightmare.

But.

Someone had thrown rolled and rubber-banded sheets of hot-pink paper up each driveway. Did taking one count as theft? Unfurled, it was a gardener's photocopied advertisement: *Call Jesus Martinez for trimming & hauling!* Those houses had huge gardens. Mission half accomplished. Thank you, Jesus.

On past outings, chalk and crayons and even charcoal briquettes have pinch-hit for pens and pencils. Not today. The asphalt and concrete looked sanitized.

Hello, what's this?

A glint.

A paper clip.

Which cannot apply pigment, but when the clip is unbent, its sharp tip incises. This, too, is writing. Consider cuneiform.

And so, I wrote. Inscribed, invisibly.

Later, at home, Jesus' paper held up to the light yielded its secrets.

Victory.

IMPROVISATION activates all of your resources: material, mental, and physical. As many scavengers are pack rats, we often already own a likely substitute for whatever we lack. We will not have the perfect thing, but we are in the habit of finding stuff free or cheap and thinking: this might be handy someday. Check us out. Pickapeppa Sauce, guitar-shaped cake pan, lug wrench, rolls of carpet, half-price theater coupons with no expiration date.

Handy. Someday.

Scavengers know what else will work. Dandelion-green salad, stapled hem.

We are inventors.

We are engineers.

We are our own resources.

EVERY DAY IS INDEPENDENCE DAY

Self-reliance is rebellion, whether we feel like rebels or not. Consumer culture does not want us to be self-reliant. It pretends it does. It talks a good game about freedom and democracy. But no: For all the truth and beauty in those concepts, which indeed abound more in America than anywhere, our powers-that-be would prefer us weak. Dependent. Desperate for product, bought at full price. They want us querulous, slavering, slack-jawed, cash and credit cards in hand, seeking instant solutions at the first sign of trouble, hunger, or thirst. *Want-get.*

Consumer culture wants consumers to imagine themselves free and democratic, decisive and bold. Consumer culture teaches that flavored coffee is creativity. Consumer culture teaches that independence means home-delivered DVDs. Up to a point, it is. A tiny, calculated creativity comprising elements designed and sold by corporations. A deceptive short-leashed independence based on your ability to buy. The rest of you is largely missing from the picture. What passes for creativity and independence in most of consumer culture is like shading in preprinted shapes in coloring books as opposed to drawing. Consumer culture has been paved and processed too long to let consumers act like pioneers, igniting fires with flint and bonding broken cups with pinesap. Nor would most even want to. The further we go from the pioneer experience, from mandatory nonstop self-reliance, the pleasanter life becomes, but also potentially the more meaningless. Pampered want-get consumers become drones, sometimes self-satisfied and sometimes depressed without knowing why. The further they go from the pioneer experience, the less they think, do, learn, stretch, reach. The less consumers know about surprise, suspense, and faith, the less they know themselves.

The more they abdicate.

CONSUMER CULTURE is a shiny, sparkly, whirling, waste-producing, world-engulfing, pick-your-favorite-product fusillade at hyperspeed, nonstop.

We wish not to participate. Except to follow, gathering detritus in its wake.

We might look like standard consumers, but no: We are fringe-dwellers, bottom-feeders, inhabiting the realm of never-knowing. Offbeat revelers and rescuers out here among the lost and the abandoned and the trashed, the designated worthless that we pluck and scrub and sometimes love.

We know what is worth what.

IN NOT CHOOSING, we choose a lot.

CHAPTER 2

IN THE BEGINNING

The Evolution of Scavenging

THE WILDEBEEST LIES DEAD AND ALMOST ENTIRELY intact, probably hit by a passing Jeep. In the dry grass, its sharp horns curve toward each other like a pair of sickles. Under an African sun, the black hide stretches sleek and taut—and too tough for the vultures, which huff and fluff around it looking for all the world like grouchy old men, necks jutting forward.

"There he goes for the bunghole," says the guide and, sure enough, the biggest bird plunges its bill into the carcass's rectum and pulls. The others join in, ruby heads jerking in, out, in, out, tearing the flesh for better access. Their black shoulder feathers spike and shirr, their hooded eyes intent. They are designed well for the job: strong legs, long talons, S-shaped heads, and necks perfect for ducking between bones and into skulls and, as now, disemboweling dead things from the inside out.

———

Vulture. Rat. Cockroach. Worm.

What do you see: A list of animals? Or a list of *insults*?

Well, it's both. These animals' names *are* insults when applied to humans.

Now take this list: Lion. Eagle. Tiger. Again, a list of animals, but in this case they're not insults at all.

What's the difference? Lions and eagles are predators—cool and efficient killing machines that stalk, slay, and then eat their victims. And yet for reasons that are not immediately apparent, humankind views this behavior as admirable. But whom did a vulture or a cockroach ever hurt? No one. It is because vultures, cockroaches, rats, worms, and thousands of other species are *scavengers* that they're reviled. Hated, even. Scavengers don't kill to eat. They eat what's already dead. They eat no-longer-living matter that has been discarded or ignored by the rest of the animal kingdom. They eat what other animals don't want. Yet despite being completely harmless to their fellow living creatures, scavengers are the most loathed species in the animal kingdom. Anthropomorphized, they epitomize the most despicable traits.

It's one of humankind's oldest and most intractable prejudices. But why did it arise? And is there any hope of resurrecting the reputation of scavengers—both animal *and* human?

The only way to find out is to go back to the beginning.

YOU ARE WHAT YOU EAT

Biologists have many ways of classifying all the life forms that inhabit this planet. Depending on your point of view, you can think of life in terms of plants/animals, invertebrates/vertebrates, terrestrial/aquatic, sentient/nonsentient, or dozens of other more precise and detailed taxonomic schema. What we're concerned with in this section are what we'll call "dietary behaviors," specifically those of animals. The two key questions are:

What is eaten?

How is it obtained?

FIRST, we'll look at *what*. Almost every species can be placed into one of four categories:

Carnivores: animals that eat (fresh) meat.

Herbivores: animals that eat plants.

Detritivores: animals that eat "detritus"—dead or decomposing organic matter.

Omnivores: animals that can eat meat, plants, *and* detritus.

Human beings are omnivores. Forget about all the claims by nutritional hoaxsters and fad-diet authors who insist variously that humans are either natural hunters who should eat only meat or (alternately) built to be peaceful vegetarians. *Not.* You can tell by our biological structures (which are altered neither by fads nor by wishful thinking) that we have evolved to be omnivores: we have canine teeth for tearing flesh *and* molars for grinding plant fiber. More important, our intestines can extract nutrition from meat, vegetables, grains, fruit—almost anything.

Now, these pedestrian details about our teeth and guts might appear unremarkable at first glance. But in fact, species possessing sharp canines *and* flat molars and multipurpose intestines are comparatively rare. Most species have highly specialized dietary behaviors and capacities. Herbivores can eat *only* plants: they have *only* grinding-type teeth to crush the plants, and stomachs and intestines that have evolved to digest plant matter and nothing else. Herbivores lack the capacity to derive much nutrition from meat, even if they were to try eating it. And the reverse is true for most predators: they have mouths full of pointy sharp teeth good for tearing flesh but not fibrous plants, and intestinal tracts that can properly digest only flesh. (That's why it's never wise to feed potato chips to the cat.) Detritivores such as millipedes, earthworms, and dung beetles can eat only food that is already decomposing. They find "fresh" food indigestible.

Omnivores, by contrast, have the amazing ability to eat, chew, digest, and extract nutrition from just about anything. In fact, that's one of the ways science identifies an omnivorous species: not necessarily by its observed behavior but rather by its biological capacity to obtain and extract nutrition from a wide variety of sources: plants and animals, living or dead matter, fresh or rotting. If you can handle all that—you're an omnivore.

Not many creatures share this nearly miraculous, highly useful survival skill. Chimpanzees, our closest relatives, are omnivores, as are pigs and chickens (which is one of the reasons both became popular as farm animals: they're easy to feed and will eat nearly anything), raccoons, crows, rats, cockroaches, pigeons, and seagulls (which explains why all of these species have thrived in the garbage-swollen urban environment), and a smattering of other lizards, birds, and fish (including, strangely, the piranha, which will settle for aquatic plants when not devouring swimmers).

NEXT, let's look at the other half of the equation: classifying animals by *how* they obtain their food. The four basic categories are:

Predators: animals that hunt, kill, and eat other living animals.

Grazers: animals that eat (living) plants.

Scavengers: animals that eat plants *and* animals that are in
most cases already dead.

Parasites: animals that derive sustenance from other living
animals without killing them.

Of course, these are generalized meta-categories, and subsumed
within them are a plethora of more specific eating strategies.
Some aquatic "predators," for example, are "filter feeders" that
don't actually hunt individual prey but rather just open their
mouths, suck in water at random, and then filter out microscopic
animals as they expel the water. Some grazers nibble off the tops
of grass stalks, letting the plant live and regenerate, whereas others tear the grass or plants from the ground, killing them as they
eat. Many of the most familiar grazers (cows, sheep, and so forth)
are "ruminants," herbivores with multiple stomachs, who chew
their food twice. However, not all grazers are ruminants. Some
scavengers eat only carrion (dead flesh), while others eat only
decaying plant matter—and so on. There are many ways to divide
up the animal kingdom, but for the sake of this particular discussion these four meta-categories will do.

WHEN YOU compare the two lists above, you'll notice correla-
tions between them. Specifically: Most carnivores are predators.
Most herbivores are grazers. *And most omnivores are scavengers.* In
fact, it's pretty difficult to think of *any* omnivorous species that
isn't also a scavenger species. Basically, an omnivore is any animal
that will eat whatever it can find. And *whatever it can find* inevitably entails scavenging.

(Note: When discussing biology, it's not wise to use the terms "always," "never," "universally," "all," and other absolutes. There are usually exceptions, and eccentric variations, and whole categories of creatures that violate any supposed "rule" about the way animals are classified or described. Hence, some predators that appear to be exclusive meat eaters will resort to eating plants on occasion; some species are carnivorous during one phase of their life cycle and vegetarian during a different stage: for example, a bug-eating caterpillar that becomes a nectar-drinking butterfly. And not *all* omnivores are scavengers nor are *all* scavengers omnivores. But we can safely say *most* are.)

In zoological terms, there are actually two different definitions of "scavenger." The first and more restrictive meaning refers to any creature that specifically eats carrion—the carcass of an animal that either has already been killed by a predator or has died of natural causes. The second, more generalized definition refers to any creature that eats discarded, abandoned, or unwanted organic matter—carrion *and* vegetation alike. In this chapter, we are using the second definition.

SO WHAT'S THE POINT? Only this: that stripped of all culture and any romantic notions about ourselves, *human beings are omnivorous scavengers*, biologically, just as we are mammals and just as we are bipedal and just as we engage in sexual reproduction and just as we sleep at night. We are scavengers, and we might as well get used to that fact.

As mentioned above, chimpanzees are far and away our closest genetic relatives, and they share most physical, biological, and behavioral traits with our species, *Homo sapiens*. And we know without question that chimps are omnivorous scavengers, using all possible avenues to acquire food. This fact alone lends support to the notion that humans must therefore be omnivorous scavengers, too, since closely related animals almost invariably have nearly identical feeding and dietary behaviors: witness gazelles and antelopes, hawks and eagles, dogs and wolves, and so on.

SELF-LOATHING

We wouldn't be going to such lengths to confirm the obvious except for the point made at the beginning of this chapter: despite the fact that we ourselves are scavengers, for some reason we regard *other* scavenger species as the lowliest, most loathsome, and even immoral creatures on earth.

How sensible is that?

We're also bipedal mammals, yet we don't think all other bipedal creatures, such as flamingos and kangaroos, are particularly loathsome. Nor do we think of all mammals as being fit for the exterminator. Of all our attributes, why do we specifically select scavenging as the one of which we are the most ashamed? Yes, there are other aspects of human nature and human biology that we often try to repress or overcome. Human sexuality, to choose the most obvious example, suffers much manipulation in many cultures. However, even the most sexually repressed cultures admit that sexuality *exists*, and that we all have sexual urges, culturally crippled as those urges might be. With scavenging, the situation is even more extreme: most modern cultures refuse to even admit that we are scavengers to begin with. It's simply too shameful, too embarrassing.

PERHAPS WE HUMANS detest our fellow scavenger species and reject our own scavenging identity for the same reason we have traditionally tried to suppress sexuality and violence: because these instinctual attributes remind us that when push comes to shove, we are animals ourselves. Civilization amounts to the process by which humans strive to slough off their primal nature, and that means convincing ourselves, despite the evidence of our own biology, that we're not brutes and beasts after all. Moral codes such as the Ten Commandments regulate sex and violence specifically as a way to elevate mankind above the animal kingdom. Cultural historians have long focused on our attitudes toward sexuality and, to a lesser extent, violence as a barometer of how far removed from our natural state we have become. But our off-and-on suppression of the scavenging urge is an equally valid way to chart our march from savagery to civilization.

Have we become the equivalent of an overweight house cat that watches impassively as a mouse scurries by, not even bothering to chase it despite frantic neural impulses in some forgotten part of its feline brain screaming, *"Hunt!"*? If so, that's a tragedy. We need to get in touch with our true selves and start working those scavenging muscles again.

SMASHING THE "LADDER OF CREATION": THE *REAL* DARWINIAN REVOLUTION

Long before there was a theory of evolution, Aristotle and other ancient Greek thinkers arranged all living creatures into what was later called the *scala naturae*, or sometimes the "ladder of creation," which categorized animals on a hierarchical scale. Mankind was of course at the top, with other mammals just below, then birds and fish and so forth, with worms and snakes and other creatures that crawled on the ground at the bottom. Inherent in this view was the assumption that some creatures were "better" than others, or more sophisticated, or more advanced. And although the exact details of this worldview slowly shifted over the subsequent centuries, the underlying principle remained: that the various species on Earth weren't merely different from each other but possessed inherent inferiority or superiority according to various scales of moral or physical measurement.

This basic philosophy persisted pretty much unchallenged until 1859, when Darwin published his epochal *On the Origin of Species*. To this day, the general populace assumes that Darwin's main conclusion was simply this: If you go far enough back, all species are related to each other, and humans are therefore descended from the same ancestors as are monkeys and apes. And while this was indeed *one* of Darwin's main points, he proved another point that was in some ways even more revolutionary. Darwin provided evidence that evolution was not the same thing as "progress," that things do not always evolve to become stronger, smarter, faster, or bigger. As he explained it, evolution is not about *improving* as time goes on but rather *adapting* to changing environments. Sometimes that leads to species becoming smaller or slower and—yes—even dumber. Prehistoric armadillos and sloths in South America were absolutely huge, as big as Volkswagens. But when they encountered predatory felines migrating down from the newly connected North America, the larger, more lumbering species were decimated, and over time they evolved to become the smaller (and comparatively more nimble) creatures we see today. Conversely, the original ancestors of horses stood only eight inches tall and were approximately the size of Chihuahuas. Now they're among the largest mammals. The archaeopteryx, the earliest known bird, started out with a fairly large brain and was probably "smarter" than its descendants. But brains are heavy and require a lot of energy to run, and if you want to specialize in flight, a brain is only going to weigh you down. At some crucial evolutionary juncture, it became more advantageous for these "flying lizards" to be able to remain airborne longer than it was to be a little bit smarter but much heavier. And so, over the millennia, birds became "birdbrains": great at flying but terrible at thinking. The flip side of that story is of course our own, in which primitive monkeys with brains the size of walnuts evolved to become the huge-brained *Homo sapiens.*

So the notion that evolution was always progressing "forward" toward some eventual goal of physical perfection was tossed out the window. And if that's the case, there's no way to legitimately claim that the species alive today are any better (or worse) than the long-extinct species that existed millions of years ago. Furthermore, Darwin showed the absurdity in trying to claim that any existing species is "more advanced" or "more sophisticated" than any other existing species. Each type has merely adapted to survive in its own environment—nothing more, nothing less. If you haughtily imagine that you're more evolutionarily advanced than a goldfish because you can solve quadratic equations and it can't, then try switching places with the goldfish and see how long *you* can survive underwater in a murky backyard pond. The point is that, yes, the goldfish can't do what you can do, but neither can you do what the goldfish does.

The main result of Darwin's illusion-shattering masterwork was to smash the ancient Greeks' ladder of creation. We are *not* on the top rung nor are snakes on the bottom rung. In fact, there are no rungs. Life is not a hierarchical system. Darwin displaced humans from their self-defined position at the pinnacle of creation. And it was this that so upset the Victorians along with almost everyone since. It's not simply that we are descended from apes and are animals ourselves; it's that our species is not really any more special than any other species. This idea is pretty hard for humans to handle. We need to feel special. We need to feel superior to other creatures. Even many scientifically minded modern evolutionists, who freely accept that we're related to monkeys, and that *Homo sapiens* are merely a type of intelligent ape, still assume deep down inside that although we are animals, we're the gosh-darned best animals of all.

What's the connection between all this and scavenging? Well, if we can't make moral judgments about the superiority or inferiority of animal physiognomy, then we can't make moral judgments about animal behavior, either. Predation is no more "advanced" or "better" than grazing or scavenging, any more than flying is more "advanced" or "better" than walking or swimming (or thinking). They're just different ways of being—nothing more, nothing less. Our social histories, our cultures, and our *prejudices* tell us that there is a hierarchy of dietary behaviors, with predation at the top and scavenging somewhere near the bottom. But evolutionary theory begs to differ. There is no scientific basis to our low opinion of scavenging. Evolutionary theory says it's just as silly to scoff at scavenging as it is to scoff at a zebra's stripes.

THE UGLY MYTH

The antiscavenging prejudice even affects our notion of beauty. For purely subjective and frankly baseless reasons, we tend to regard predators as attractive and scavengers as ugly. Pop quiz: Which do you think is more beautiful—an eagle or a vulture? A lion or a hyena? *But,* you argue, *it's not that I admire predators because they hunt; I admire them for their skills.* Really? Cheetahs are fast—but pound for pound, considering their size, cockroaches run faster. Do you admire the cockroach for *its* speed? Will you name your track team the Roaches?

Nope.

Scavengers are perceived as ugly merely because humans have traditionally disapproved of their behavior. Our opinion of how they look is determined by how they acquire food and eat.

Pretty is as pretty does.

Then again, not every scavenger species gets a bad rap. Many are viewed neutrally—for instance, bluejays, catfish, ants, jackals, and buzzards. A very few even have *positive* reputations: for instance, ravens (because they're supposedly the most intelligent birds) and raccoons (because they're cute). Conversely, some scavengers have bad reputations only because of *other* attributes, not because of their feeding behavior: many species of wasps are scavengers, for example, but humans hate them because of their painful stings, not because they scrounge for fallen fruit and rotting meat. Despite the rare exceptions, humans hate scavenger species *in general*. The reason some species escape derision is that humans just don't know much about their eating strategies. (Catfish are scavengers? Who knew?)

FOOD WEBS

Modern biologists now look at the world in terms of "food webs." A food web is essentially the same thing as an ecosystem, but it focuses specifically on what eats what. Originally, these dietary relationships were viewed more simplistically as a series of ever more powerful predators dining upon one another: a blade of grass "eats" sunlight through photosynthesis; an ant will then carry away and eat a kernel of grain from the grass; a spider will catch the ant and eat it; a praying mantis will eat the spider; a rat will eat the praying mantis; a snake will eat the rat; a mongoose will eat the snake; and a hawk will then swoop down and eat the mongoose. All very neat and tidy. But the closer we look at how things work in the real world (as opposed to a diagram in a book), the more we see that reality is much messier. A mongoose will eat the meat of a snake, but it won't eat the large bones or the head. Who eats those? The ant might eat the grain, but who eats the dead stalk of grass at the end of the season? And everything that goes into a mouth comes out the other end as excreta: as nauseating as it may be to ask, who eats that?

It turns out the missing factor that transformed incomplete theoretical food chains into fully realized food *webs* was (you guessed it) scavenging. Scavengers, once narrowly classified as animals that feed only on carrion, were redefined as any creatures that seek out and consume nonliving organic matter. That would include carrion (the carcasses of dead animals), dead plants or parts of plants (fallen fruit, dry grass, rotting wood), detritus (decomposing material), feces and other secretions (*blech*—but we gotta be honest), and any leftover bits. Once scavengers were added to the mix, it became readily apparent that nothing in nature went to waste; everybody's got to eat *something*, and eventually everything and everyone is eaten by something or somebody else. Round and round the biomass goes; the organic molecules that constitute the substance of all living things are endlessly recycled from body to body to soil, from soil to plant to another body to soil to fungus to soil to another body to another body, endlessly. The authors of Genesis got it partly right when they wrote "for dust thou art, and unto dust shalt thou return"—but that's just scratching the surface, because once you've returned to "dust" (or soil or detritus, as we'd now call it), your molecules are bound to eventually reanimate once more as a lawn or a gopher or a narwhal or all three. The Earth has only so much organic material, and it's constantly being reused as the building blocks of life.

And scavenging is an essential component of this biomass life cycle. Without scavengers to eat and decompose all the dead stuff, the planet would eventually become a vast cemetery of inedible dead animals and dead plants, the nutrients therein bound up and lost forever. The global ecosystem would collapse, or become severely degraded, without scavengers busily fulfilling their crucial role. And yet humans have inexplicably condemned scavengers as unnecessary, unclean, and unwanted. Perhaps if all the globe's scavengers—animal and human—went on strike for a week, the rest of the ungrateful world would learn how important scavengers really are.

A WORLD WITHOUT SCAVENGERS WOULDN'T BE MUCH OF A WORLD AT ALL

Scavenging animals are nature's recyclers and cleanup crews. And the same holds true for human scavengers. Society tends to negatively associate scavengers with garbage, but the scavengers don't *create* the garbage—instead, they get rid of it, or process it, or diminish it, or turn it into something useful. Scavenger species play a key role in nearly every ecosystem. Despite how much humans have historically loathed scavengers, we need scavengers.

The *world* needs scavengers.

On a grander scale, the entire planet's habitability depends to some extent on scavengers. When you get right down to it, the very soil under our feet is worm shit. And these worms are detritivorous scavengers, eating the dead rotting plants that nobody else wants. In fact, long after Charles Darwin was already famous for developing his epochal theory of evolution, he spent years writing his last book, *The Formation of Vegetable Mould Through the Action of Worms*, which was exclusively about earthworms and how they have completely transformed the Earth. "I doubt whether there are many other animals which have played so important a part in the history of the world," Darwin wrote, referring specifically to how all the planet's topsoil—which is what we now call what he called "vegetable mould"—came from earthworms that had chewed up and excreted scavenged food. And without topsoil there could be very little terrestrial plant life; and without plant life, very little animal life, and so on.

Not only is the Earth's arable soil a gift from scavengers, but our climate is partly a gift from scavengers as well. Because of the global-warming controversy, the average person thinks of "greenhouse gases" as a problem that needs to be solved. But without *any* greenhouse gases, we'd all freeze to death. By trapping radiant heat in our atmosphere, greenhouse gases have modulated and warmed the Earth's climate for hundreds of millions of years and created the temperate climate necessary for life to flourish. Yet the atmospheric balance is very delicate, which is why just a tiny increase in greenhouse gases can cause a rise in temperatures. Historically, the three main natural greenhouse gases have always been carbon dioxide, nitrous oxide, and methane. Without the exact proportions of these three gases in the atmosphere, the Earth would become icebound. Of the three, methane in particular is partly a by-product of a scavenger species: termites. And a significant portion of the Earth's methane comes from—to put it bluntly—termite farts.

Termites are one of those interesting scavenger species that are *not* omnivorous: they're specialized scavengers, eating only wood—usually in the form of dead and fallen trees that are ignored and unwanted because no other species can eat them. Only the termite has the unique ability to scavenge, eat, and digest this otherwise inedible material, deriving nutrition from wood cells and then farting out methane as a sort of accidental by-product. Now, termites are tiny, and each termite doesn't produce much methane, but scholars estimate that there are well over 200 quadrillion termites on Earth at any given time, and they've all been farting twenty-four hours a day for at least 65 million years; and the primary result is that these scavengers have warmed up the planet enough for the rest of us to feel comfortable.

Both worms and termites are aided in their planet-wide eco-system alteration by specialized microbes, the tiniest scavengers of them all, which live symbiotically in the intestinal tracts of worms and termites and digest and break down plant fibers that otherwise would be bound up and lost to the ecosystem forever. Without termites and their microbes, the Earth would have long ago become a barren, frigid petrified forest of fallen trees, since there would have been no way for the organic material in the wood to be recycled back into the ecosystem—were it not for the liberating digestive tract of the termite.

PARASITES

For all our passionate defense of scavengers, another category of creatures has an even worse reputation: parasites.

As mentioned above, the names of individual scavenger spe-cies, such as vulture and rat, are considered insults—yet the word "scavenger" itself has no strong negative connotations. Calling someone a scavenger will not provoke a fistfight. But just try call-ing someone a "parasite." Then duck.

Many people can't discern the functional difference between scavengers and parasites. The two are often conflated in the public mind. But the distinction is significant. A parasite is any organism that habitually takes nutrients from the *living* body of a "host," almost always damaging the host's health or fitness in the process, without actually killing it. (Technically speaking, a parasite must live permanently *on* or *in* a single host, though some scientists consider this definition overly restrictive, and prefer to classify organisms such as mosquitoes to be parasites, too; we'll be using the looser definition here.) In this sense, we see parasitism as being similar to theft, when viewed from a human moral framework, since the parasite "steals" nutrients and health from the unhappy host. Scavengers, by contrast, do not steal food but rather take only what has already been discarded or what is unclaimed and unwanted.

Unfortunately, as with most things in the animal world, the distinction is not as self-evident as we're making it out to be—and it is this blurring between parasitic and scavenging behaviors that is partly to blame for the bad rap that scavengers have gotten throughout history.

WHAT IS OWNERSHIP?

It's not always obvious what counts as unclaimed in nature. If you find an acorn on the ground, it might appear to you to be an unwanted acorn, but for all you know a squirrel put it there for later retrieval while he's off gathering more acorns; and if you were to carry away the acorn, you'd unwittingly make the transition from "scavenger" to "thief." But this same principle often holds true in reverse: even though as *Homo sapiens* we understand what counts as "ownership" within human culture, and why we put things where we do, such distinctions are entirely lost on other scavenger species.

Take, for example, the origins of the relationship between rats and humans. Evidence suggests that rats first were attracted to human settlements to eat the abundant grain to be found in early agricultural societies. Harvesting back then was terribly ineffi-cient: some of the stalks were inevitably left unharvested in the field, and the seeds would often fall to the ground during trans-port or threshing. That left a tasty buffet for scavenging species such as rats.

The whole purpose behind growing and harvesting plants during the warm season was to save them up and have enough to survive through the barren winter. Hence, much of the grain that humans collected ended up in storehouses, which, in those days, were neither airtight nor ratproof. A storehouse was just a big, inviting pile of grain waiting to be eaten.

Now look at this situation from the rat's point of view. A rat knows nothing about the concept of ownership and probably very little about foresight and planning ahead. If it sees some food on the ground, it eats it. Simple as that. The rat is not making moral assessments: "Before I eat this grain of wheat, I ask myself, who *owns* it?" No. To a rat, there is absolutely no difference between grain it finds scattered in an autumn field and grain it finds in a rectangular wooden enclosure that humans call a storehouse. For all the rat knows, we put the grain there for the purpose of later discarding it. Maybe the storehouse is actually our garbage dump. So the rat slips into the storehouse and eats our winter supplies without the slightest guilt or awareness that he's doing anything wrong. He's just scavenging for food as he does every day. He remains blissfully unaware that we humans regard him as a thief who "steals" something that we imagine is our possession.

It is this subtle misunderstanding (and countless similar mis-understandings) that is partly responsible for the bad reputation that scavengers have in the human moral framework. Though the scavenging animal is just doing what it naturally does, we see it as a criminal wickedly violating our societal norms. So that when people engage in scavenging behavior, they are tarred with the same brush as the rat and the cockroach—even though the human scavengers (one hopes) aren't actually stealing anything. But because their behavior is *reminiscent* of animal scavenger behavior, and because animals *don't* understand that they're violating a "rule," the human scavengers become outcasts even though they are not themselves lawbreakers.

(That said, there are always a small percentage of human scavengers who intentionally or not cross the line and scavenge things that aren't necessarily free for the scavenging. When someone does that, they *have* graduated from scavenger to thief, since—unlike the rat—they are all too aware of their moral transgression. Be sure to pay attention to Chapter 9, "The Scavenger Code of Ethics," which examines the line between true scavenging and conscious theft.)

As a consequence of this interspecies misapprehension, early humans conflated scavengers and parasites: a mosquito surreptitiously steals our blood, which we need to survive; a rat surreptitiously steals our grain, which we also need to survive. What's the difference?

AGGRESSIVE SCAVENGING

Further complicating matters is the fact that some animals do indeed engage in what we might call "aggressive scavenging." And here is where our thesis comes close to falling apart. As noted above, animals and their behaviors cannot be so conveniently placed into a series of distinct categories. Behaviors comprise a long spectrum—a messy, ugly, and sometimes embarrassing spectrum. So how to explain away these "aggressive scavengers," animals that sometimes use violence to steal food from other animals that can rightfully claim prior ownership?

Take hyenas, for example, which are partly scavengers in that they often dine on carrion—dead animal flesh. When a group of hyenas comes across the carcass of an animal that has died of natural causes, they'll merrily start eating it since no one else seems to want it. But hyenas are not always lucky enough to find dinner just lying on the ground. Often, it's much easier to simply hover around on the periphery when a predator makes its kill. That way, the scavengers don't depend wholly on chance to find their food; they'll just let the predator do the shopping and slaughtering for them.

After a predator has taken down its prey, the *polite* hyenas will patiently wait for the predator to eat its fill, and move in only when it has abandoned the remaining carcass. But hunger and politesse are often at odds. And most hyenas are, frankly, not very polite to begin with. Hungry hyenas will often start aggressively harassing a predator as soon as it's had its first bite. And sometimes they'll succeed, driving away a cheetah or leopard from its kill and stealing the carcass for themselves. (Lions, however, usually fight back against hyenas.)

It would be too facile to say, "Such vile behaviors simply don't count as scavenging in my book." Hyenas are in some ways the prototypical scavengers, and "stealing" food through harassment or violence was in fact the very activity that originally defined scavenging as a zoological category.

But as it turns out, this type of behavior seems mostly limited to those species—such as hyenas and jackals—that are "predator-scavengers." Hyenas will scavenge, but only when it's convenient. Just as often, if not more often, they are traditional predators as well, chasing down and killing living prey, usually in large packs.

Predator-scavengers are killers, and because of this they have no compunction about using violence to get what they want.

At this level in the food web, distinctions blur. For example, lions, which are considered *the* model predator, will in fact sometimes turn the tables on aggressive predator-scavenger species such as hyenas and steal carcasses from them as well, reversing what we imagined were their traditional roles. Upon closer inspection, there is not much substantive difference between the food-obtaining behaviors of "pure" predators such as lions and predator-scavengers such as hyenas: both species primarily hunt, both will steal carrion from rivals, and both will have carrion stolen from them. The difference is merely in matters of degree—how commonplace is each behavior, a few percentage points this way or that. Hence, lions could also be classified as predator-scavengers, or hyenas could be classified simply as predators; it's really just a matter of linguistics and labels.

But this blurry line between the two groups contributes substantially to our historical perception of scavengers as "immoral," because species that we traditionally considered scavengers were observed stealing food that belonged to others—food that these animals *knew* belonged to others, and that they wrested away by force. The problem is that this has always been somewhat of a misperception, because this observed thievery was really just the actions of a predator in an aggressive scavenging mode—and predators always use violence or the threat of violence, even when scavenging. The truth is, *most* species that we think of as either pure predators or as exclusively aggressive scavengers merely occupy some hard-to-pin-down point on the predation-scavenging spectrum, and there is no distinct biological or behavioral line dividing the two concepts.

The first step toward reviving the reputation of human scavengers is to revive the reputation of the animal scavengers that gave the behavior its bad name in the first place. And once we recognize that "admirable" lions and "nasty" hyenas essentially obtain their food in the same way—sometimes hunting, sometimes stealing—then we can see that it makes no sense to idolize lions and disparage hyenas, nor to maintain a prejudice that favors predators over scavengers.

So the next time you hear about *The Lion King*, ask yourself: Why isn't it *The Hyena King*?

PARASITOIDS

Believe it or not, there's even a zoological category that, when judged by human sensibilities, ranks *beneath* parasite: the "parasitoid," a type of creature whose feeding behavior is considered so shockingly evil (for lack of a better term) that even Charles Darwin himself felt that parasitoids were the most loathsome of all animals, and that a sane God couldn't possibly have purposely designed something so horrible—which therefore lent support to his theory of naturally occurring evolution. Parasitoid behavior is often used as the model for fictional monsters in science-fiction films, horror stories, and urban legends.

Like ordinary parasites, parasitoids derive their nutrition from the bodies of still-living animals. The difference is that parasitoids inevitably eat their hosts to death, usually from the inside out. The most famous real-world parasitoid is the ichneumon wasp, which was partly the inspiration for the life cycle of the extraterrestrial creature in the *Alien* film series. Ichneumons and other parasitoids generally lay their eggs in the bodies of another animal (often, though not always, another insect), using long needlelike "ovipositors" which look like stingers but are actually sexual organs that function similar to a mosquito's proboscis. After an interspecies "reverse rape," in which the female ichneumon wasp jabs its ovipositor into an unwitting victim, the eggs hatch inside the host's body and start eating. Immature ichneumons have evolved to grow entirely *inside* other species' bodies. At first, the host is not terribly inconvenienced by the tiny larval ichneumons nibbling away in its body, but eventually the ichneumons grow big enough to start what must be an agonizing process of eating their adoptive godparent from the inside out. Finally, the mature ichneumons will "hatch" from the hollowed-out corpse of their host, and the cycle begins anew.

You can see why, after studying them, Darwin commented, "I cannot persuade myself that a beneficent and omnipotent God would have designedly created the Ichneumonidae with the express intention of their feeding within the living bodies of Caterpillars."

Compared with parasitoids, scavengers seem positively saintly.

THERE'S NOTHING WE WON'T EAT

Earlier in this chapter, we saw how scavenging is an inborn genetic trait in our species, something we can't disavow any more than a panda could deny that it likes eating bamboo shoots. And while we do possess that trait, it's only part of the story; human beings are uniquely complicated, and (depending on the circumstances) we can and do fill *every* trophic role in the global ecosystem: predator, grazer, scavenger—even parasite. Early humans were what we now call "hunter-gatherers," which is simply another name for "predator-scavengers." We hunted and ate animals but also scavenged for fallen fruit and whatever else the local environment provided. Later, with the development of agriculture, some humans became full-time grazers as well, because that's what agriculture really is: organized grazing on an industrial scale. And yes, we occasionally engage in parasitical behavior, too, though it is comparatively rare. East African tribes cut open bulls' necks to drink their blood, then let them heal—similar to the strategies of mosquitoes and vampire bats, which both count as parasites under the term's informal definition. Also, "bleeding" maple trees for syrup and rubber trees for sap is parasitic behavior on our part, since we injure and extract material from a living thing without killing it. This is typical of omnivores, who not only eat anything and everything but seek out food in every possible way.

ABANDONING PREJUDICE

When you finally throw off the stigma of a long-standing prejudice, the subconscious urge is to seek revenge—to reverse the roles and place yourself at the top of the hierarchy. But, joyful as it might feel for us scavengers to emerge, blinking, into the light of social acceptance, we should not now spoil the moment by creating a new prejudice against those who formerly loathed us. Because there is an uncomfortable truth that we should always keep in mind: as scavengers, we are to a certain extent dependent on the wastefulness of top-tier predators. This is true in the animal world as well as in its human analogue. Vultures don't kill anything themselves; they need the lions to not only do the killing for them but to also abandon the unwanted remains after they're done eating. And without big spenders tossing out their old couches and coffee tables after buying this year's latest models, what would human street scavengers have to scavenge? Yes, a small number of vultures could survive on animals that died of natural causes, and urban scavengers could satisfy themselves solely with what was lost accidentally; but the pickings would be mighty slim in both cases. This isn't to say that we should *admire* the wasters: only that we should just admit we are in a mutually beneficial symbiotic relationship with them. Perhaps there is no way to avoid an undercurrent of mutual disdain—we hate them for wasting, they hate us for scavenging—but we are eternally bound together in a marriage of necessity.

HUMANS EVOLVED to be scavengers—and yet we've also taught ourselves to hate scavenging. And therein lies the source of the problem. Because try as we might to distance ourselves from our animalistic scavenging roots, this is not a trait we can choose to eliminate at will. And this fact contributes to our species-wide self-loathing and self-denial.

Wouldn't you rather just Dumpster-dive?

CHAPTER 3

THE OLDEST PROFESSION

The Rise and Fall of a Prejudice

IN CHARLES DICKENS'S NOVEL *BLEAK HOUSE*, THE rag-and-bone man named Mr. Krook is "short, cadaverous, and withered, with his head sunk sideways," his head and throat "gnarled with veins and puckered skin." Signs on his window read BONES BOUGHT and WASTE-PAPER BOUGHT and LADIES' AND GENTLEMEN'S WARDROBES BOUGHT. Dirty bottles frame the doorway of his filthy warren, on whose floor loll "second-hand bags," bundles of women's hair, and a "litter of rags." He is, we learn, "a dealer in cat-skins among other general matters." Greeted by Krook, whose thin hands are "like a vampire's wings," the narrator "naturally drew back."

Naturally.

Such scenes have been repeated in art and literature countless times: the scavenger as physically foul and psychically sinister.

For millennia, the loathing that humans have felt for scavenger animals has extended to human scavengers as well. From hunter-gatherers to ragpickers to Untouchables to junkmen to Dumpster divers and beyond, human scavengers have traditionally been relegated to the lowest social rungs. In this chapter we'll probe the reasons for this revulsion—tracing how society has scorned and shunned scavengers from prehistoric times onward—and we'll offer a glimmer of hope that this prejudice is finally beginning to disappear.

AT WHAT POINT did early hominids stop being animals and start being humans?

Of course there are those who insist that we're *still* nothing more than animals, and, conversely, those who insist that mankind was recently created out of thin air in the image of God. But the mainstream contemporary view is that sometime in the far-distant past, our primordial ancestors were some kind of animal; and that now, as humans, we have a "soul" or at least an ineffable spark of self-awareness that marks us as distinct from every other organism on the planet. What marked the transition from one state to the other? What distinguished that "evolutionary Adam" from his apelike parents?

IT'S A DIFFICULT QUESTION, one that has bedeviled our greatest thinkers and philosophers since earliest recorded history. And while the answers have been many and varied, a common thread through them is this: that it is not our biology but our *behavior* that distinguishes us from other creatures. "What is a man, if his chief good and market of his time be but to sleep and feed? A beast, no more," wrote William Shakespeare in *Hamlet*, encapsulating a long-standing view that persists to this day: first, the assumption that being akin to an animal is a bad thing; and second, that *acting* like an animal, and doing the things that animals do, is what brings us down to the level of beasts. Hamlet listed spending all day sleeping and feeding as distinctly animal-like, but there are more specific animal behaviors that are forbidden by our civilized social mores, and it is these prohibitions that make us human. First: Don't kill indiscriminately, the way animals do. Second: Don't have sex indiscriminately, as animals often do. In short: Resist our animal urges, our animalistic nature.

As discussed in the previous chapter, one of our basic evolutionary traits as humans is the urge to scavenge. And although the prohibition against scavenging is not usually spelled out in humankind's various religious texts and philosophical treatises, neither are other basic animal behaviors explicitly discouraged or prohibited, even though we know to avoid them anyway: don't deposit feces and urine at random whenever you get the urge; don't run around naked, and so on. Over time, in almost every corner of the world, a generalized credo arose: the less you act like an animal, the better. While that has long been noted by social historians, what has not been noted is that scavenging counts as "acting like an animal" too, since it is one of our basic instincts, one shared by many of our fellow omnivores. And this is partly at the root of why scavengers have been shunned by human society since the dawn of recorded history, just as have killers, adulterers, and thieves: because their behaviors (and scavenging) make us "no better than beasts."

So the answer to the question posed earlier in this chapter, many would say, is that we started becoming humans when we made the conscious decision to stop acting like animals. And that includes our species-wide consensus to pretty much stop scavenging. Remember that the earliest *Homo sapiens* 200,000 years ago were biologically almost indistinguishable from modern man; yet those early humans, many would say, were not quite humans at all, since they still lived like animals and acted like animals and showed little if any evidence of complex thought. Hovering in the background behind our society's inchoate disapproval of scavenging is the vague feeling that *if you scavenge, you risk losing your soul.* Because it's not the shape of your body that makes you a human being, but the nature of your behavior. Which means: Stop that scavenging and get a job.

HUNTERS AND GATHERERS

Precivilizational humans were nomadic, often following game animals as they migrated, or moving from one area to another during different seasons in search of food. Those tribes lucky enough to live in tropical areas with sources of nutrition available year-round usually stayed in one region permanently. But in the vast majority of early hunter-gatherer societies, one constant appears virtually universal: men did most or all of the hunting, and women did most or all of the gathering. And in this context, "gathering" is just a euphemism for "scavenging": collecting fallen fruit, finding and digging up edible roots and tubers, gleaning berries, collecting firewood, garnering seeds or wild grain, and so on.

This hunter-gatherer lifestyle continued for thousands and thousands of years, so it's easy to see how scavenging—the "gatherer" half of the equation—became associated with women's work, since women were the gatherers. When some human populations began transitioning to agriculture around twelve thousand years ago, gathering was replaced by farming, which men and women did equally. This shift was not instantaneous: agriculturalists and hunter-gatherers lived side by side for millennia, often competing for land and resources. Over time, the agriculturalists became ascendant and drove the hunter-gatherers into the mountains and forests and other peripheral areas. Xenophobia against the hunter-gatherers arose as farmers and, later, city dwellers looked down on them as primitive and backward.

This prejudice also manifested as derision toward anyone who *acted* like those "primitives." And although hunting continued to be practiced by farmers and urbanites, scavenging for its own sake was for the most part abandoned—scorned as "women's work," effeminate, too reminiscent of the hungry, dirty, bad old days. And so this, too, was a contributing factor to the growing bias that was held against scavenging in male-dominated societies: scavengers were like animals, scavengers were like primitives, and scavengers were like women. Scavenging was effeminate. And that made it inferior.

Thus a deep-seated prejudice against scavenging became part of human culture around the world and endured throughout history, up to the present day.

This ancient bias is still with us, as we lug around anachronistic cultural baggage from one epoch to the next. But at this stage in human development, what purpose does this prejudice serve anymore? We in the modern world no longer compete for resources with spear-wielding hunter-gatherers. We no longer look down on "women's work" as inherently substandard or less valued. We no longer try to pretend that we don't have evolutionary traits that connect us to our mammalian relatives. The fundamental rationale for our rejection of scavenging has long since expired. The time has come to put the baggage down, to unburden ourselves of unnecessary self-loathing (which is what anti-scavenging feelings essentially are, since we *are* scavengers whether we accept it or not), and move forward with a light step and a lighter footprint.

And roomy pockets for toting whatever we find.

THE MORAL CODIFICATION
OF ANTISCAVENGER BIAS

The collection of books we now call the Old Testament has for thousands of years been one of the cornerstones of Judeo-Christian civilization, the original font of the moral philosophy upon which so much of the Western worldview is based. And of those Old Testament books, the most important one in many ways is the first: Genesis, which spells out our culture's creation myths. And right there near the beginning of Genesis we find a primal rejection of the migratory hunter-gatherer lifestyle—and by extension, scavenging.

Because this is so key to our understanding of the anti-scavenging bias, let's examine the passage in full. The New King James Version translates Genesis 4 thus (with relevant passages in italics):

Now Adam knew Eve his wife, and she conceived and bore Cain, and said, "I have acquired a man from the LORD." Then she bore again, this time his brother Abel. Now Abel was a keeper of sheep, but *Cain was a tiller of the ground*. And in the process of time it came to pass that Cain brought an offering of the fruit of the ground to the LORD. Abel also brought of the firstborn of his flock and of their fat. And the LORD respected Abel and his offering, but He did not respect Cain and his offering. And Cain was very angry, and his countenance fell.

So the LORD said to Cain, "Why are you angry? And why has your countenance fallen? If you do well, will you not be accepted? And if you do not do well, sin lies at the door. And its desire is for you, but you should rule over it."

Now Cain talked with Abel his brother; and it came to pass, when they were in the field, that Cain rose up against Abel his brother and killed him.

Then the LORD said to Cain, "Where is Abel your brother?"

He said, "I do not know. Am I my brother's keeper?"

And He said, "What have you done? The voice of your brother's blood cries out to Me from the ground. So now you are cursed from the earth, which has opened its mouth to receive your brother's blood from your hand. *When you till the ground, it shall no longer yield its strength to you. A fugitive and a vagabond you shall be on the earth.*"

And Cain said to the LORD, "My punishment is greater than I can bear! Surely You have driven me out this day from the face of the ground; I shall be hidden from Your face; *I shall be a fugitive and a vagabond on the earth,* and it will happen that anyone who finds me will kill me."

And the LORD said to him, "Therefore, whoever kills Cain, vengeance shall be taken on him sevenfold." And the LORD set a mark on Cain, lest anyone finding him should kill him.

Then *Cain went out from the presence of the LORD and dwelt in the land of Nod on the east of Eden.*

Now, these lines, needless to say, are among the most famous ever written. And they've been analyzed countless times from countless points of view. But for our purposes, let's adjust the lens and look at Genesis 4 from a scavenging perspective.

Adam was the first human being, but he was sort of a wild man, living naked in nature until he was banished by God. However, his first son, Cain, was "a tiller of the ground," meaning that he was the Bible's first nonmigratory agriculturalist, the original farmer. Cain represents our transition from savagery to civilization, from being merely *biologically* human, as was Adam, to being *behaviorally* human.

But after discovering that Cain has committed a grievous sin, how does God punish him? By sentencing him to once again become a "vagabond on the earth," for whom the ground "shall no longer yield" crops. In other words, God punishes Cain by forcing him to become a migratory hunter-gatherer, wandering forever in search of food and a place to rest, since he is no longer allowed to grow crops. Turned into a scavenger—the worst punishment of all.

Because of modern linguistic confusion, the phrase "land of Nod on the east of Eden" is now often mistaken to mean a place of dreams, where you "nod off" to sleep. But it actually has nothing to do with slumber. In this setting, "Nod" comes from the Hebrew word for "wandering." Thus the phrase "dwelt in the land of Nod" is really just a poetic way of saying, "lived a migratory lifestyle." There was no actual place called Nod.

We can see from Genesis that, even at the very dawn of our culture, having a stable agricultural life was the preferred state of being, and the worst thing that could happen to you was having to subsist as a scavenger. Thousands of years' worth of Judeo-Christians ask: If God says so, who are we to argue? Even in our civilization's founding myth, scavenging is regarded as a curse. How can we escape a prejudice *that* deep?

CASTES AND OUTCASTS

Social hierarchies are an inescapable feature of human culture. Nearly every society or civilization that has ever been studied has official or unofficial social classes based on wealth or tradition or profession or race or religion or some unknown factor lost in the mists of time. Yet a common feature shared by most of those at the bottoms of hierarchies, wherever in the world they happen to be, is that they end up living as scavengers. The only mystery is: Were scavengers assigned the lowest social status merely because they were scavengers to begin with—or did people trapped by birth in low social standing become scavengers because no other employment was open to them? Either way, all around the world, scavenging is traditionally associated with the lowest rung of society.

India's caste system is perhaps the best known of all hierarchical social systems; and even though it was officially abolished when India became an independent nation, old customs die hard and many of the caste-based prejudices live on today. The lowest caste are known in English as "Untouchables." (There is a drive to replace that term with a name that doesn't sound like such a put-down: some prefer the word "Dalit." But other such alternatives have come and gone, and the term "Dalit" is still not universally used, so it's not clear if it will ever become the "official" name for this caste. For now, we'll stick with "Untouchables.") In his 1935 novel *Untouchable,* Mulk Raj Anand—now known as "India's Charles Dickens"—revealed the shocking treatment allotted to these pariahs. While sweeping up trash in a temple's courtyard, the hero Bakha is startled by the congregation, who at the very sight of him shout, "Polluted, polluted, polluted," and surge away to escape his contaminating presence. "A thumping crowd of worshippers rushed out of the temple," Anand writes. Among them is the priest, a Brahmin who leads the chant "Polluted, polluted, polluted!" as a larger and larger crowd "took the cue and shouted after him, waving their hands, some in fear, others in anger, but all in a terrible orgy of excitement." One member of the crowd can be heard above the others:

"Get off the steps, you scavenger! Off with you! You have defiled our whole service! You have defiled our temple! Now we will have to pay for the purification ceremony. Get down, get away, you dog!" Adds another: "A temple can be polluted according to the Holy Books by a low-caste man coming within sixty-nine yards of it, and here he was actually on the steps, at the door. We are ruined."

The reason Untouchables were given their unflattering sobriquet is that they were once legally forbidden to touch anyone of a different caste. This rule was so severe that even the *shadow* of an Untouchable was considered taboo, as was the ground he or she had walked on and objects he or she had handled. Why? Untouchables were considered irrevocably unclean, both hygienically and ritually, because of their occupations, which often involved death, discards—and scavenging. Untouchable groups typically worked cleaning up roadkill and other dead animals, carting away the carcasses of dead cows, the carrion of which they would eat before making the hide into leather. They also worked as street cleaners, toilet cleaners, and garbage collectors, picking through other people's discards for usable material. Some present-day Untouchables live in or near dumps, scavenging for recyclables. Though scavenging is not universal among Untouchable occupations, it is a fairly common feature and raises the question: Over time, did the scavenging professions become classified as the lowest caste? Or was Untouchability an inherited social rank-

ing, and if you were born within it you had no choice but to engage in the kind of work higher castes refused to do? It's a
chicken-or-egg conundrum that probably has no definitive answer. Most likely the two options coexisted simultaneously and
worked in tandem to create a mutually reinforcing social loop
from which there was no escape.

A sect of Hindu ascetics known as the Aghori voluntarily scavenge human corpses floating down the Ganges, drag them
ashore—and eat the rotting flesh. They also drink from human
skulls and sometimes even eat animal droppings that they find.
You might think this disproves the theory that *all* cultures have a
negative outlook toward scavenging. But it actually confirms the
theory even more: the Aghori don't do these things because they
are proscavenging. Quite the opposite. They believe that the fast-
est way to achieve enlightenment is to intentionally violate the
most forbidden Hindu taboos, to consciously reject all social customs. So they purposely engage in the most extreme scavenging
behavior *because* it is the most unacceptable possible lifestyle. The
Aghori's bizarre customs only serve to prove that scavenging
ranks as the *least* acceptable occupation in India.

JAPAN ONCE had its own version of the Untouchable caste,
though it is much less known around the world than India's
version. The *burakumin* (sometimes called just *buraku* or, in early
Japanese history, *eta*) comprised a virtual parallel society in medieval Japan, living in segregated villages and performing many of
the same tasks as India's Untouchables—dealing with corpses,
dead animals, cleaning and garbage collection, ragpicking, and
begging. For centuries, the government officially discriminated
against them, effectively rendering the *burakumin* a permanent

underclass who were in part scavengers. In this case it was Shinto customs, not Hindu theology, that marked them as ritually impure. Even though the discriminatory laws were lifted in 1871, when Japan entered the modern era, lingering revulsion and distrust of *burakumin* remain to this day in Japan, where worried parents sometimes hire private investigators to find out whether their children's prospective spouses have *buraku* ancestors—which would still be considered a shameful mark on the family heritage.

And so it was in other societies around the world. Although most hierarchies were not as clearly delineated as the official systems in Japan and India, it remained true that most cultures were stratified, and that scavengers, where they existed, were at or near the bottom rung of society. But there were reasons for this other than prejudice. Keep in mind that prior to the industrial era, and the mass production that came with it, scavenging was necessarily a subsistence occupation. It was pretty much impossible to become wealthy, or even economically comfortable, as a scavenger. Until recently, scavenging was a do-or-die lifestyle, not a hobby or a choice, as it is for many of us in the modern world. Medieval ragpickers in Europe scavenged discarded clothing to resell in order to gain a few coins to buy food and survive; by contrast, the ragpickers of twenty-first-century America for the most part prowl flea markets and thrift shops searching for funky decor and cool cheap clothes—by choice and for fun. In the modern world, we have endless seas of manufactured goods to pluck through. In the pre–mass production, preindustrial era, objects were all made individually. Thus each object was considered precious and less likely to be discarded. Scavengers faced slim pickings in those days, which is why only the most impoverished resorted to scavenging—and why it was almost always only a survival tactic.

THERE WERE of course exceptions to the negative cultural associations toward scavenging. The ancient Egyptians worshipped deities that were the personifications of scavenger animals. Anubis, god of the afterlife, was a jackal. Nekhebet, goddess of rebirth, had a vulture as her totem animal. Khepri, the sun god, was depicted as a dung beetle. So did ancient Egyptians have an entire scavenging-themed religion? Actually, no. Most of their other deities were associated with animals that *weren't* scavengers: Hathor was a cow, Bastet a cat, Wadjet a cobra, Sekhmet a lioness, and so on. The Egyptians didn't uniquely worship scavengers to the exclusion of everything else; the best that can be said is that they had no prejudice *against* these animals, which at least put them one step ahead of other cultures in tolerating scavengers. The reasons for this are not entirely clear. Perhaps because the Egyptians lived in harsh desert conditions where scavenging animals are a more prominent part of the visible ecosystem, the local people became more accustomed to them.

GLEANING

"Gleaning" is not a word you hear much these days, but in early agricultural societies, gleaning was one of the primary forms of scavenging, and sometimes served as an important social-welfare mechanism by which the poor survived. Ancient Jewish society in particular observed this custom, and it was even spelled out as an inviolable law in Leviticus 19:

> And when ye reap the harvest of your land, thou shalt not
> wholly reap the corner of thy field, neither shalt thou gather

the gleaning of thy harvest. And thou shalt not glean thy vineyard, neither shalt thou gather the fallen fruit of thy vineyard; thou shalt leave them for the poor and for the stranger: I am the LORD your God.

Deuteronomy 24 spells out a similar prohibition:

When you reap your harvest in your field and have forgotten a sheaf in the field, you shall not go back to get it; it shall be for the alien, for the orphan, and for the widow, in order that the LORD your God may bless you in all the work of your hands. When you beat your olive tree, you shall not go over the boughs again; it shall be for the alien, for the orphan, and for the widow. When you gather the grapes of your vineyard, you shall not go over it again; it shall be for the alien, for the orphan, and for the widow. You shall remember that you were a slave in the land of Egypt; therefore I am commanding you to do this thing.

In other words, farmers and orchardists and vintners were forbidden to harvest their fields thoroughly, and were expected to leave unharvested vegetables, grains, and fruit for poor scavengers to come along and "glean"—which means to gather unwanted and forgotten farm produce at the end of the season for personal use. The system is taken to the extreme every seventh year, known as the *shmita*, or "sabbatical year," during which *all* produce is to remain unharvested and left for scavengers to collect for free. This system to some extent is still observed today by religious farmers in modern Israel, though many have found the antiquated law too financially burdensome, and various mechanisms have arisen to sidestep it—such as temporarily selling one's land to someone else every seventh year.

Through these ancient Jewish gleaning laws, we can see that scavenging was recognized by the ancient Hebrews as a significant survival strategy for the downtrodden. These biblical regulations are among the very few *pro*scavenging laws of the premodern era.

UNBUILDING EMPIRES

Few people who travel today through Italy and Greece to admire the ancient ruins realize that they are seeing the handiwork of scavengers—or, to be more precise, their destructive handiwork. The ancient Romans, in their heyday, went on a centuries-long building spree covering much of Europe with impressive structures made of marble, stone, and cement. When the Roman Empire fell, Europe descended into the so-called Dark Ages. At that time, there was no longer any central government to maintain the thousands of public buildings, aqueducts, city walls, and temples. Most of these buildings would have survived intact through the millennia were it not for local scavengers, who treated them essentially as quarries, ancient Home Depots, handy hardware stores for free construction materials. The most visible example, Rome's Colosseum, was never damaged in war. The only reason it isn't in better condition today is that over the centuries, bit by bit, scavengers broke off loose parts of the structure or carted off stones loosened by earthquakes to use as the building materials for their own homes. The same is true with nearly every ancient ruin you see in Europe.

Medieval scavengers unbuilt the glorious empires of ancient Greece and Rome.

ON THE ROCKS

One of the most notorious of historical scavenging lifestyles is that of the "wreckers." Made famous by Daphne du Maurier's *Jamaica Inn*, wreckers were a class of professional beachcombers who lived in various coastal regions but most famously in Cornwall and Scotland. Starting in the seventeenth century, Great Britain became a global maritime power, and ships of all sorts were constantly coming and going in and out of British ports. But the British coastline was famously treacherous, and in the era before radar and GPS and foghorns, ships would frequently run aground or get dashed on the rocks—particularly in Cornwall and Scotland. Their cargo was often so valuable that local fisherfolk opportunistically turned to scavenging the washed-up wreckage at every opportunity. The villainous Cornish characters in du Maurier's story took it a step further, intentionally *causing* shipwrecks by displaying deceptive lights on- and offshore, luring treasure-laden ships to their doom. Though this tale was fictional, it is thought to be based on factual incidents. In her 2005 book about maritime scavenging, *The Wreckers*, Bella Bathurst calls them "pro-active beachcombers."

At their worst, these wreckers were rumored to deliberately let crew and passengers drown in order to gain unimpeded access to those unfortunates' possessions and the ships' cargo. Over the years, such shocking stories inflamed the negative public perception of beachcombing scavengers in the English-speaking world. Although modern technology makes it impossible to trick ships into wrecking, and although former wrecker communities have turned to fishing and tourism for their livelihood, we still get occasional glimpses of how it once must have been. In January 2007, the container ship *MSC Napoli* partly sank and then ran aground off the southern English coast. More than one hundred of its gargantuan shipping containers fell into the English Channel and shortly thereafter began washing up on beaches in Devon. Within a matter of hours, word spread across the region that an astounding variety of new consumer goods was being strewn in massive quantities along the shoreline. The BBC reported: "Over the last two days scavengers have descended on the beach, taking away goods that included BMW motorbikes, wine, face cream and nappies," as well as barrels of liquor, shoes, hair-care products, steering wheels, exhaust pipes, gearboxes, foreign-language bibles, and much more. The BBC also noted that a nearly forgotten law especially created to stop the wrecker subculture in earlier centuries was cited to halt the frenzy: "The 'despicable' behaviour of scavengers has forced the authorities to invoke ancient legislation to stop raids on cargo on a Devon beach. Powers not used for 100 years will be used to force people to return goods recovered from the stricken container ship *MSC Napoli*." Despite the legal threat, most of the modern-day wreckers escaped with their booty undetected.

RAGPICKERS AND JUNKMEN

After the Diaspora, when Jews were compelled by circumstance to live in countries where they were tiny minorities, they were often forbidden to practice most trades and ended up in unpopular professions such as money lending and tax collection. But those positions were open only to Jews who were somewhat well educated and could demonstrate business acumen. A substantial number of lower-class Jews ended up becoming itinerant scavengers—known as rag-and-bone men in England, *strazzaroli* (or *stracciaroli*) in Italy, and so on. Today the generic term "ragpicker" is often used, but such scavengers were not always limited to just rags. As Dickens showed us in *Bleak House*, rag-and-bone men would collect households' leftover bones to be sold to glue factories; they also collected scrap iron and lead to be melted down, rags and discarded clothes to resell or to be shredded and made into paper or second-generation fabric, and hair to be made into wigs. And more: they also collected bottles, animal skins, paper, and anything else that could be recycled or repaired.

In his memoir *The Old Home Town*, Izhak Ze'ev Jonis describes the Polish shtetl of his youth, where in the yard of a leather tanner

lived the rag-pickers with their wives, children, horses and carts. When the farmers' field work ended, the peddling season began. The old rag-picker Avrum Hersch, and his sons, Shmuel, Meyer Nusen, Michael and Yerahmiel, as well as his sons-in-law, Aron, Menashe and Elia, each set out on a different road with wagons laden with all sorts of goods. They carried chinaware, plates with floral designs, pots, glass beads of various colors, decorative pins made of tin resembling gold, buttons, needles, thread, safety pins and many other items. These would cause farmers and their wives eagerly to search every nook and cranny of their homes for scraps of iron, rags, bones, copper and brass. Trade with the village was based on barter. The rag-pickers paid with the pretty items they brought with them from town [where they had scavenged them from wealthier districts]. For many years the shacks [of the scavengers] were full of old rags, iron and other metals, and bones. Women and children with red, pus-encrusted eyes, skin covered with boils and with swollen bellies, ran back and forth rummaging through these piles and sorting them out.

Needless to say, ragpickers in whatever country, Jewish or not, were considered the bottom of the social pecking order.

They were a common sight in poor New York neighborhoods such as the Lower East Side, where an entire underclass of impoverished scavengers scoured the urban landscape for anything of value. In *How the Other Half Lives*, his book about New York City slums, the social reformer/photographer Jacob Riis included his now famous 1888 photograph "Home of an Italian Ragpicker." It shows an exhausted-looking woman with a baby in her lap, hemmed in by barrels, buckets, and what look like overstuffed duffel bags. Her mouth is turned down at the corners and her eyes gaze upward, as if seeking relief. Italian immigrants were then the city's main scavengers, Riis wrote:

There is money in New York's ash-barrel [that is, trash barrel] but it was left to the genius of the *padrone* to develop the full resources of the mine that has become the exclusive preserve of the Italian immigrant. Only a few years ago, when rag-picking was carried on in a desultory and irresponsible sort of way, the city hired gangs of men to trim the ash-scows before they were sent out to sea. The trimming consisted in levelling out the dirt as it was dumped from the carts, so that the scow might be evenly loaded. The men were paid a dollar and a half a day, kept what they found that was worth having, and allowed the swarms of Italians who hung about the dumps to do the heavy work for them, letting them have their pick of the loads for their trouble. To-day Italians contract for the work . . . sorting out the bones, rags, tin cans and other waste that are found in the ashes and form the staples of their trade and their sources of revenue. . . . Whenever the back of the sanitary police is turned, he will make his home in the filthy burrows where he works by day, sleeping and eating his meals under the dump, on the edge of slimy depths and amid surroundings full of unutterable horror. The city did not bargain to house, though it is content to board, him so long as he can make the ash-barrels yield the food to keep him alive, and a vigorous campaign is carried on at intervals against these unlicensed dump settlements; but the temptation of having to pay no rent is too strong, and they are driven from one dump only to find lodgement under another a few blocks farther up or down the river. The fiercest warfare is waged over the patronage of the dumps by rival factions.

Although the profession slowly died out and/or transitioned to "junkman" by the middle of the twentieth century, the prejudice remained. The 1950 Academy Award–nominated comedy film *Born Yesterday* featured as lead characters a boorish nouveau riche millionaire and his uneducated girlfriend arriving in Washington, D.C., to bribe politicians. The girlfriend eventually wises up and turns the tables on her blustery beau, but much of the comedy derives from the supposedly hilarious fact that the corrupt millionaire made his fortune as a junkyard owner. The very idea that a junk dealer could become a millionaire social climber sent audiences across America into hysterical laughter. Could anything be more absurd? Everyone knows junkmen are the scum of society; how ridiculous to show one becoming rich off his junk! Naturally the scriptwriters depicted the junkman millionaire as monstrous, greedy, and sneaky.

Naturally.

ALTHOUGH professional scavengers have mostly vanished from Western societies, they still abound in many Third World countries, where they focus on modern-day recyclables such as plastic bottles. Now, as ever, they occupy the lowest socioeconomic rung and endure persecution—often motivated by the general public's revulsion at the mere sight of them. Typical was a new law that took effect in Indonesia's capital, Jakarta, in 2008, doubling the penalties against scavenging. Under the new law, scavengers—*just for being scavengers*—could be rounded up, arrested, and jailed for up to two months or forced to pay a fine of up to 20 million rupiah. That's the equivalent of around $2,100. The average scavenger earns the equivalent of $2 a day. To enforce the new law, the number of "public order agents" deployed to apprehend scavengers quadrupled.

"There's no other job for me but to be a scavenger," a homeless Sumatran immigrant told an Agence France-Presse reporter soon after the law took effect. "What I earn today is only enough to buy food. There's nothing left for renting a room." While his wife and toddler slept in a wood-and-tin cart, the Sumatran slept on a mat. By day he collected cardboard, paper, and plastic cups. "Nobody wants to lead this kind of life," he told the reporter. "But it's far better than being a loser like a beggar. It's more shameful—they don't have any pride or make an effort in life."

Another scavenger described her humiliation upon having been arrested:

"My cart was demolished in front of me," she recalled. After spending her prison sentence being forced to work in the garden of a government office, she fled back to Jakarta as soon as she could, she told the reporter, preferring her freedom as a scavenger. She specialized in scavenging the refuse left behind after parties. "I love a party," she told the reporter. "If any house has a party, I just wait there outside until the party is over to pick up the garbage."

THE GOLD RUSH: SCAVENGING HYSTERIA

While urban nineteenth-century America still looked down on scavenging, at the same time on the wild frontier it was a different matter altogether. Having arrived with only whatever essentials they had been able to transport via covered wagon, frontier dwellers were compelled to constantly improvise.

Frontier-style scavenging went into overdrive in 1848.

While building a sawmill on the American River in California, a local man named James Marshall found a few yellow pebbles under the clear water. After a few quick tests confirmed that the pebbles were actually gold nuggets, the news immediately spread to his workmen and others in the vicinity. Marshall allowed them to go scavenging for nuggets themselves in the river. The first few months were delirious: nuggets could be had for the taking. Just poking around on the riverbed or in adjoining creeks yielded nuggets galore. Poor laborers became wealthy in a matter of days.

Within months word had reached the outside world, and the California Gold Rush was on. Much has been written about the forty-niners, who descended on California from every corner of the world in 1849 by the tens of thousands looking for quick riches. But the smart ones were in fact the forty-eighters—those who went looking for gold in 1848, before that huge crush of humanity arrived. The forty-eighters had it easy because they were the scavengers: the gold was just lying around, waiting to be picked up. In fact it was this detail that caused the California Gold Rush in the first place. What attracted the hordes wasn't merely the news that gold had been discovered, but that it could be scavenged effortlessly. Plenty of other places had gold, but it was hard to find and harder to extract. What made California's gold so attractive was that all you had to do was bend down and pick it up. Or so the rumors went. And went and went—from Scandinavia to Chile to China. Sailors heading around Cape Horn sang a chantey:

Blow, boys, blow, for Californ-i-o . . .
Oh, there's plenty of gold, so I've been told,
On the banks of the Sacramento.

Soon enough, all the surface nuggets had been found. Then prospectors took it to the next level, scavenging more aggressively by "gold panning"—that is, digging under the mud at the bottom of the creek beds and sifting out the nuggets in the flowing water. It took a bit more effort, but it was still scavenging, a comparatively easy way to accumulate riches. But after the main wave of forty-niners arrived and swarmed over the landscape, even the panning opportunities diminished sharply. Within a couple of years, California's gold was scavenged out. By the early 1850s, new arrivals began engaging in more extreme and labor-intensive methods—diverting entire rivers, washing away hillsides with high-powered water jets, and eventually following the gold back to its source in the mother lode, where the only way to get at it was with pickaxes and dynamite. This wasn't scavenging anymore. This wasn't fun anymore. This was *work*. Lured by tales of easily scavenged gold, countless treasure seekers arrived over the following decade and ended up doing hard labor for little recompense.

In a letter to her sister back east, a pioneer described her cobbled-together California home: "The fireplace is built of stones and mud. . . . The mantel piece—remember that on this portion of a great building, some artists, by their exquisite workmanship, have become world-renowned—is formed of a beam of wood, covered with strips of tin procured from cans, upon which still remain in black hieroglyphics, the names of the different eatables which they formerly contained." The letter writer, who had grown up in a plush home, now joked: "How shall I ever be able to content myself to live in a decent, proper, well-behaved house, where toilet tables are toilet tables, and not an ingenious combination of trunk and claret cases, where lanterns are not broken bottles, book cases are not candle boxes, and trunks not wash stands." With very little available for sale—and with just about everything besides beans priced sky-high—pioneers scavenged for food as well, gathering wild berries and brewing tea from foraged mint and mock "coffee" from ground acorns. Of course, they hunted wild game as well.

The old prejudice against scavenging vanished on the frontier since everyone was doing it.

Nonetheless, the California Gold Rush transformed American culture. It not only populated the American West, but it also did a lot to raise the reputation of scavenging. The notion of being able to simply *find* treasure sitting on the ground if you look diligently enough still lingers in the American psyche. Some say it fuels the characteristic American optimism, the spirit of adventure that spawns latter-day "gold rushes" such as the dot-com boom.

THE GREAT DEPRESSION

They say that once you learn how to ride a bicycle, you never forget. Prompted to ride again after decades spent never touching a bike, you suddenly find yourself pedaling like a triathlete before you even realize you're doing it.

It's the same way with scavenging. Say you've never scavenged before in your life. Say you've *always* enjoyed the comforts of consumer retail culture as far back as you can remember. But then—uh-oh!—circumstances change. Suddenly you're homeless, say. Suddenly you're starving. Suddenly you're poor. Desperation takes over, and those scavenger skills that our species acquired over millions of years of evolution—and which you've never accessed even once before in your life—automatically kick in.

That's what happened on a wide scale in the early 1930s when the Great Depression plunged millions of ordinary people in Western nations into harrowing poverty. For years, Americans had been steadily moving away from scavenging as an occupation. By 1928, it was practically erased from the collective memory. Then suddenly . . .

Times of crisis restart—and kick-start—the scavenging instinct. History has shown again and again how wars and disasters turn even the laziest, most shopping-addicted consumers overnight into foragers. At such times, anyone who is already a scavenger or who possesses scavenging skills such as vigilance and tolerance is way ahead of the game. But when survival is at stake, everyone scavenges.

During the Great Depression, tens of thousands of displaced and newly homeless people gathered together for protection and created scavenger settlements. Nicknamed "Hoovervilles" after then President Herbert Hoover, these shantytowns sprang up from coast to coast, from Central Park and Brooklyn to Seattle's tidal flats, comprising shacks made of rocks, scrap metal, lumber, cardboard, and wooden crates. Scavenged newspaper used as bedding was dubbed "Hoover blankets," and "Hoover leather" was scrap cardboard placed inside shoes whose soles were worn through. Hooverville dwellers ate food scavenged from wherever it could be found, which was usually urban trash cans. At its height, Seattle's Hooverville had more than two hundred shacks, housing unemployed World War I veterans and laborers from the failed fishing, logging, and construction industries. The shape and state of each shack depended on the skills of the scavenger who had built it. Archival photographs of the Seattle settlement—which stood on the grounds of a former shipyard a few blocks south of what is now Pioneer Square—show tidy, slant-roofed scrap cottages as well as slapdash asymmetrical shelters whose doorways are gaping rough-edged holes. A resident of Pittsburgh described his local Hooverville as "one of the most unusual sights we've ever seen in any city. Here you will find men living in home-made 'houses' constructed of box wood and lumber, begging description. Many curious folks come out to 'Shantytown' and a guide eagerly shows one around with explanations as to who is who and what is what in 'Shantytown.' Any donation you may give is part of the community chest and shared by all the dwellers." In the 1936 film *My Man Godfrey*, nominated for six Academy Awards, a wealthy young socialite on a "scavenger hunt" ventures into a Hooverville and meets an actual scavenger—whom she aims to bring home. The camera pans the dark city dump where tumbledown shacks perch against slopes of garbage. Smoke rises from a cook fire around which we see derelicts warming themselves.

Whether or not they lived in Hoovervilles, new population sectors emerged during the Great Depression. The suddenly unemployed homeless American eager to work—to do any chore or job—in exchange for goods, food, or money was known as a hobo. But any suddenly unemployed American *not* eager to work, who relied instead on scavenging, became known as a tramp or a bum. Making the rounds in those days was a folk song called "Hallelujah, I'm a Bum," which went in part:

Oh, why don't you work
Like other men do?

How the hell can I work
When the skies are so blue?

Taking its title from the song, the 1933 film *Hallelujah, I'm a Bum* stars Al Jolson as Bumper, the unofficial mayor of New York City's bums, who with his African-American sidekick Acorn presides over a group of charismatic scavengers who frankly admit that they'd rather scavenge than work. One can only wonder how the truly poor—who couldn't afford cinema tickets anyway—felt about this slap-happy musical in which a Marxist trash collector nicknamed Egghead exults about the coming revolution, and Jolson sings a song titled "What Do You Want with Money?" Made during the stark depths of the Depression, the film actually celebrates the scavenging lifestyle, portraying bums as jolly and genuine, even heroic: Bumper saves a suicidal woman from drowning herself in Central Park. For all its grit and squalor, these bums prefer their rough-edged authentic lifestyle to the slick duplicity and daily grind of the "straight" world. Tellingly, the film is sometimes screened with the alternative title *Happy Go Lucky*.

Even those whom the Depression didn't render homeless and jobless had to learn how to scavenge. Throughout their lives, the parents of both of the authors of this book have told stories about their youths spent scrounging, saving, recycling, and reusing: about sheets of newspaper and writing paper used over and over for various purposes, about hand-me-down clothes collected from better-off relatives, about old sweaters unraveled so that the yarn could be knitted into socks, mittens, and more. Learned in childhood, such practices turned out to be lifelong lessons not just in terms of survival but also of philosophy. Like those who live through wars and natural disasters, those who suffered through the Depression learned to scavenge but also learned to transcend shame. They learned the value, literal and figurative, of money not spent. "Save your pennies," Anneli's Aunt Bessie—who died in Florida in 2006, aged ninety-three—used to advise, "and your dollars will take care of themselves." Heard enough times, such maxims sink in. Although both of us were raised in middle-class environments, both of us are and have always been scavengers because Depression-era values were passed down to us.

As un-PC as it sounds, living through the Depression ended up *raising* our forebears' self-esteem, because all that scrimping and saving made them realize that they could survive under any circumstances. Suddenly straddling the bicycle of necessity before they could even doubt themselves, they were riding like the wind.

SCAVENGERS-BY-CIRCUMSTANCE continue to surface during crises of all kinds. During the 1992–1996 siege of Sarajevo by Bosnian Serbs, many urbane Sarajevans were seen collecting firewood and foraging in dumps and trash containers.

Will a day come when that crisis befalls your town, your family, you? How would you build *your* Hooverville?

THE *ACTUAL* OLDEST PROFESSION

Deep down inside, we remain scavengers at heart, scavengers in our genes. Scavenging, not prostitution, is the oldest profession. As recently as a few decades ago, the public viewed with admiration the rugged miner who dug iron ore from the ground to make steel—yet the same public eyed with pity and disgust the homeless tramp who collected cans to resell for pennies a pound at the scrap yard. But really, we now realize en masse, the miner and the tramp do exactly the same thing. Both provide us with the raw materials for steel. Cans *are* ore. As we stride now into what is proving to be the "Recycling Century," it's hard to imagine on what basis anyone ever imagined that the miner was morally superior to the can collector. And can it be that the prejudice has already started to swing the other way? The miner, many might say now, despoils the environment, whereas the can collector cleans up our garbage. But again, we should be wary of substituting one prejudice for another. Unless we are willing to revert to anarcho-primitivism, living wild in the woods, we must always remind ourselves that the raw material of civilization has to come from *somewhere*, and without the miners of the world and the lumberjacks and the farmers and the factories, we'd have nothing to scavenge to begin with. The time has come to treat scavengers as equals.

And equal is good enough for us.

CHAPTER 4

SCAVENOMICS

Nothing Is Garbage Anymore

ONE DICTIONARY'S DEFINITION OF ECONOMICS IS: "the study of the production, distribution, and consumption of goods and services."

Notice anything missing? What happens *after* "consumption"? Traditional economic theory has glossed over this bothersome detail for centuries. Once the product, whatever it is, successfully reaches the hands of the consumer, its economic journey was deemed complete. Man buys product, man takes product home, family utilizes product. The end.

But reality is messy and not so simple. Will that consumer utilize that product forever, until the end of time? Of course not. Eventually, in five minutes or fifty years, the product will become used up, or broken, or obsolete, or outdated, or its owner will die, or any number of other eventualities could occur whose result is that the object ends up in the trash.

And then?

Welcome to the world of scavenomics.

Scavenomics picks up where economics traditionally leaves off. It is the study of that *other* half of the cycle that has been so conveniently ignored by economists: What happens to goods *after* consumption, and how do they find their way back to "production" at the beginning of the cycle?

Scavengers, naturally, are the prime driving force for this hidden half of the story. We are the ones who take society's trash and either *reuse* it, introducing it back into the *middle* of the standard economic system (trash rechristened as goods for distribution and consumption), or *recycle* it, introducing the material back at the *starting point* of the system (trash reprocessed into raw material for production). Scavenomics thereby becomes the corrective to a field of study that has heretofore been off-balance, and which until recently has examined only half the available information.

Modern economic theory is not as blind as it used to be. These days recycling is regarded as a valid economic activity, as yet another way to make money. (Reusing and repurposing, however, are pretty much still off the radar screen.) But to the extent that it's been considered at all by economists, scavenging is regarded as a behavioral *problem*, a sort of consumer dysfunction that prevents people from properly purchasing and consuming their fair share of stuff. If too many people scavenge instead of buying retail, then the economy won't grow and everything will head into a recession. Which, needless to say, makes economists unhappy. But the reverse can also be bad: mindless, endless overproduction, overconsumption, and then overdisposal. Scavenging as a naturally occurring method of acquisition puts the brakes on what otherwise might be a runaway train of capitalism; by opting out of the consumer cycle, we slow the system down to a reasonable pace.

And it's no accident that scavenging serves this function.

It's an example of the "invisible hand" posited by early econo-mist Adam Smith, which was his way of articulating that eco-nomic systems naturally structure themselves to be as efficient and self-regulating as possible. His "invisible hand" metaphor was actually much the same thing as Darwin's "natural selec-tion": animals, species, people, systems, decisions, and attitudes adapt to changing environments, to maximize their chances for success. That "invisible hand" is none other than evolution at work—but in an economic system as opposed to a natural environment.

It goes like this: If there is overproduction, and everybody buys too much stuff, then sooner or later some of that stuff will be discarded; and if enough gets discarded, then people will see that the products they used to pay for can now be acquired for free through scavenging; and once a sufficient number of people become scavengers, they stop buying new stuff, and production will thereby slow down to sustainable levels. The opposite is also true: If *everybody* starts scavenging, then production will cease entirely because no one is buying; but if nothing is being pro-duced, then the inventory of scavengeable material will eventu-ally disappear and there will once again be a demand for new stuff, and production will start up again. This process, in a nut-shell, is how scavenomics works. It's what keeps the capitalist system and the global economy in balance. When a society, such as 1980s Japan, engages in reckless overproduction and overcon-sumption, the principles of scavenomics dictate that a collapse is bound to happen; and when a society, such as contemporary sub-Saharan Africa, depends *too much* on scavenging (in this case on donated goods and food), it's also indicative of an economy that needs fixing. Scavenomics is the economics of self-regulating moderation.

IT'S NOT EASY BEING GREEN

There's a secret about waste no one really wants to talk about. And it's this: *The freedom to generate waste and not worry about what happens to it is what powers the economy.* While it might not be taboo to mention this fact, it *is* taboo to have the wrong opinion about it. And in the modern world, the wrong opinion is: Maybe that's not such a bad system. Maybe we *should* let manufacturers and entrepreneurs and individuals get away with not taking into account the full cost of their productive activity.

One of the underlying principles in contemporary "green economics" (will this fad for appending "green" before every word end soon? We can only hope) is that businesses must factor in the full expense of every single step and every single consequence of their manufacturing. While it's an interesting idea in principle, sometimes it ends up causing additional consequences and inefficiencies. That's because it forces businesses that would otherwise only have one specialized skill to have to deal with other problems they know nothing about.

TAKE, as a fictional example, a guy who comes up with a clever way to twist bicycle inner tubes into funny animal shapes. He gets so good at this that he starts a business making funny animal-shaped inflated bicycle inner tubes for birthday parties. The business becomes successful and he hires workers to twist inner tubes in assembly-line fashion. He has to order truckloads of inner tubes in bulk to satisfy the demand. During the production process, the inner tubes often pop and then have to be discarded, and some designs involve cutting the inner tubes to be shorter and discarding the remnants. The end result is that his business is now not only producing funny inner-tube animals, but also producing an awful lot of waste consisting of popped and trimmed inner tubes. Now, in the old economic model, he would just throw these away and hopefully no one would notice or care. But in the new green economy, disposing of the waste tube remnants now becomes his responsibility. He has to become an expert in rubber disposal, rubber recycling, and toxic emissions. He can no longer just throw them away—he has to *cope* with them and their consequences somehow. He has to learn a whole new skill set. It becomes burdensome to him.

Next he is informed that the rubber trees tapped to make the rubber for his funny animals suffer serious bark injuries, and that his consumption of rubber causes on average the deaths of five rubber trees every year. He is then required to fund the Rubber Tree Replacement Program, as well as the Rubber Tree Tappers Health Care System, since the workers are all getting carpal tunnel syndrome from tapping all those trees. The poor guy: all he wanted to do was make funny animals.

The moral of this (entirely fictional) story is that we're forcing a guy who knows nothing about rubber disposal and rubber plantations to now take responsibility for what happens to the waste from his business and for the consequences of his raw material consumption. Yet none of that is his specialty. All he knows how to do is twist things to make them look like funny animals. Eventually, if the regulations are too byzantine, he might just give up and throw in the towel—because the business is no longer fun or profitable once he becomes responsible for the full environmental cost of everything he does.

Multiply that scenario by thousands of times and you can see how a rigidly enforced green economy would necessarily be a less-productive economy. The upside, of course, is that there would be less pollution and less environmental degradation. Now, there are different kinds of waste, and actual *pollution* pollution such as toxic emissions should indeed be discouraged and/or paid for. But not all waste is so obviously valueless. Left out of this equation are the scavengers, who might be otherwise called "specialized waste exploiters." It is the scavengers who often discover the hidden value in what is otherwise thought to be pure waste of either no value or negative value. In the scenario above, if the entrepreneur was allowed to simply throw away his inner-tube scraps, before long a second-tier scavenging entrepreneur would discover the bins full of rubber tubing headed for the landfill, salvage them (at no cost), and come up with the idea to cut them into rings, which he can then sell as "eco-bracelets" for a dollar apiece. In this scenario, we now have two successful businesses (the funny animals and the eco-bracelets) but no waste whatsoever because the waste itself was turned into a resource. In the original scenario there was also no waste, but as a consequence there were *no* successful businesses, either.

One of the principles of scavenomics is to unleash the creative power of scavengers. Often they, and only they, can come up with a use for discards, turning negative value into positive value. A real-world example comes from the realm of chocolate production. For centuries cocoa farmers discarded as trash the husks left over from shelling the cocoa pods. But in recent years, entrepreneurial scavengers thought of selling the otherwise worthless cocoa husks as gardening mulch to Americans, who love anything that smells like chocolate (which the husks do). Now, in some gardening outlets, you can buy scavenged cocoa-husk mulch. Multiply *that* scenario by thousands of times and the power of scavenomics becomes clear.

Productive capitalism has been proven over the centuries to create the largest amount of wealth for the greatest number of people. Its formerly (though no longer) hidden flaw is that it tended to damage the environment in the process. For a very long time this inconvenient detail was shrugged off as "the price of progress." The environment has now become so damaged, however, that we're starting to think that the price might be too high. The new green economy tries to rectify this flaw with compulsory compliance and burdensome regulations. Scavenomics proposes to achieve the same desired result—less environmental destruction—using a more laissez-faire, entrepreneurial approach: give scavengers free rein and let them turn the waste into something of value.

In truth, green economics and scavenomics are not always in opposition. Often they are complementary, and scavenomics can be viewed as a subset or a variant of green economics.

THE CONSUMPTION CYCLE

The mistake comes in thinking of the global economy as a straight line, or a linear process that starts somewhere and ends somewhere better. The traditional (and unconscious) way of viewing economic activity is: Raw materials are obtained from nature, then manipulated in various ways, and then made into products for mankind's benefit. The end. But of course a key detail (which is actually more than just a detail) is glossed over. Because there is no "end"—economic activity is not a line but a circle. A continuous cycle. The missing steps are: This manufactured or refined material, whatever it might be, is eventually used up or becomes broken or obsolete or unwanted, and is then discarded. And *then* somewhere, somehow, by somebody or something, it all gets fed back into the beginning of the system and the cycle begins all over again. This can happen on a very short time scale—the product being immediately scavenged and reused or repurposed; or on a medium time scale, in which the products are broken down into their original constituents and recycled back as the raw material for manufacture; or on an extremely long time scale, in which everything is at first just unceremoniously "thrown away," which essentially means returned to the Earth far from its point of origin in a new place such as a landfill or a dump, and perhaps in a million, or ten million, or who-knows-how-many years in the future, some distant civilization of superhumans will discover a rich "deposit" of iron ore in a location formerly known as Melvin's Salvage Yard and U-Find-It Car Parts Emporium.

The goal of scavenomics is not simply to focus attention on this missing step of the economic cycle but to minimize the time frame and energy expenditure of that step. So, from a scavenomics point of view, waste disposal is the least desirable and least efficient behavior, because the raw materials contained in the trash become lost to us for an extremely long time. Recycling is one step better, because the aluminum molecules or cellulose fibers are reintroduced into the human ecosystem as raw materials fairly rapidly, with a moderate amount of energy expended. But scavenging—ah, scavenging is the gold standard of economic efficiency, or at least of this part of the economic cycle. Because when anything that is unwanted and discarded gets scavenged and reused or repurposed, it immediately reenters the global economy with practically no energy expenditure at all. It doesn't need to sit around for a million years turning to rust or topsoil; it doesn't need to be shipped to China and melted down and recast as ingots and then shipped to a factory and turned into a simulacrum of whatever it was in the first place. Without having to travel anywhere, or use any energy, the object once again becomes useful to humankind, without any processing or time wastage whatsoever. You can't get more efficient than that.

Because all economic activity is part of a cycle, it makes no logical sense that one part of the cycle—scavenging and recycling—has lower status than other parts of the cycle, such as manufacturing and consumption. Each stage is entirely dependent on all the others and should be regarded as equal. Scavengers are that portion of the cycle that converts material into something useful once it has been "excreted" by society. As mentioned in Chapter 2, without termites scavenging and digesting all the world's wood for millions of years, liberating and recycling the nutrients locked up therein, the globe would have long ago become a sterile wasteland of fossilized fallen trees; similarly, without the scavenging part of the human economic cycle, the world will eventually become one gigantic dump of unwanted and unused garbage.

Recycling *is* a form of scavenging, but contrary to popular opinion, it is not the most eco-friendly form of scavenging, nor is it a revolutionary act. Recycling is often superior to *not* recycling, certainly, when no other options are available, but it only serves to reinvigorate the consumption cycle. As far as beneficial environmental and economic behavior is concerned, scavenging unwanted items or materials and rescuing them to be used as they were originally intended to be used is far and away the most efficient. Scavenging and then *repurposing* objects is second-best, because repurposing often requires some energy and effort. And finally, and least efficient, is recycling, which requires that materials be sorted, transported, collected, sorted again, transported again, melted or processed, refined, transported again, used in manufacture, transported again, purchased, brought home, used for ten minutes—and then thrown once again into the recycling bin. All recycling does is feed more raw material (albeit comparatively eco-friendly and inexpensive raw material) back into the start of the standard consumer cycle. It doesn't disrupt or undermine that cycle in the slightest; it only helps our mass-production consumer culture grow even larger. Depending on your point of view, that can be either a good or a bad thing. Ironically, the type of people most likely to recycle are the ones who feel that mass consumption is a bad thing.

OPTING OUT

Self-sufficiency, which might be viewed as a positive attribute under most circumstances, terrifies most economists and social philosophers. For an economic system to function as a whole, and for a community to feel cohesive, everybody needs to work together, to rely on each other, and to be part of the interconnected system. But someone who is entirely self-sufficient—what role does he or she play in society? For the most part he or she is absent from the quotidian interchanges that make civilization hum. And it is this perception that has in part caused our leaders and politicians and economists and philosophers to regard scavengers—to the extent that they think about scavengers at all—with a mix of exasperation and fear. Because scavengers, more than just about any other social category, are self-sufficient. We don't really participate very much in the whole manufacture-sell-consume-dispose cycle that drives the modern world. *What's the matter with you people? Are you* trying *to make the economy collapse?*

After the 9/11 attacks caused a significant downturn in economic activity, the United States government famously encouraged people to get the country back on its feet by doing one simple act: *Shop*, we were told. Buy, buy, buy. It's your patriotic duty. And, interestingly, people *did* get back to shopping, rather quickly in historical terms. Yet they headed back into the stores not because the government told them to but rather because they

eventually felt they *needed* to; life goes on, recession or no recession. We hadn't changed our basic economic behavior—we simply
took a brief hiatus to recover from the shock. Consumers who had
been briefly stunned eventually snapped out of it and went back
to shopping.

But scavengers—we weren't shopping in the first place, even
before the recession. Our economic behavior, or lack thereof,
really doesn't appear to affect the overall economy one way or the
other. The manufacture-sell-consume-dispose cycle will keep
rolling along, whether we scavenge or not. Sure, if we somehow
managed to convert a substantial percentage of consumers to the
cult of scavengerhood, then customers for new products would
evaporate and the economy would crash. But then what? With a
collapsed capitalist economy, new products would stop being
made. Which would mean fewer products being disposed of or
entering the scavenging subeconomy. At the same time there
would be a massive new contingent of ex-consumers turned scavengers. The end result would be too many scavengers fighting
over too little stuff. Not only would scavenging then cease to be
enjoyable, but scavengers would not be able to even meet their
basic material needs. If you moved into a new place and needed
a couch, there'd be no free couches left to scavenge. So you'd end
up having to (gasp) *buy* a new one. Which means the scavengers
would eventually revert to being new-stuff consumers. And with
a new wave of customers once again demanding goods, manufacturers and retailers would naturally jump into the gap, and the
economy would be kick-started all over again.

This scenario reveals scavengers' embarrassing little secret: we
may *appear* to be self-sufficient, but we're not. Our self-sufficiency
and nonparticipation in the capitalist system are only apparent,
an optical illusion. We are deeply enmeshed in the mainstream
economy—it's just that part of the economy to which no one

really pays much attention. (Or *paid* attention; things are starting to change.) Scavengers need capitalism, and capitalism needs scavengers. Without your castoffs and junk, we'd have nothing to scavenge. And without someone removing, processing, and reintroducing materials back into the system, the capitalist economy would eventually run out of raw materials. But this relationship between the scavenging world and the consumer world is an uncomfortable one, one that both sides are ashamed to admit even exists. Scavengers fancy themselves to be rebels and revolutionaries and independent outsiders who have no use for the oppressive world of drones and squares and copycats. On the other side, capitalists and consumers don't like to think about what happens to all that stuff after it completes its journey down the manufacture-sell-consume-dispose conveyor belt. Too messy. Too inconvenient. Just sweep that detail into the, uh, trash.

RESOURCE DEPLETION AND REGENERATION

We just finished saying that the manufacture-sell-consume-dispose cycle will keep rolling along, with or without scavengers. And while that has been true so far in history, it won't remain true for long. Up until fairly recently, we've regarded planet Earth as a sort of inexhaustible source of raw materials. There was no way, it seemed, to actually run out of anything; there was always more, more, more. More wood—the forests extended off to forever. Entire continents were covered with trees. More metal—just keep digging down, down, down for more ore. More oil—it gushed up in geysers that never stopped. Underground oil fields were of seemingly incalculable size. More, more, more of just about everything.

And while our population remained comparatively small, and

our individual consumption patterns were not wildly extravagant, this perception was accurate. But two factors changed the equation: overpopulation and the global spread of the consumer culture. Very rapidly in historical terms, the number of people who demanded a possession-filled life of leisure exploded exponentially, and without warning we suddenly could feel society's spoon scraping the bottom of the Earth's once inexhaustible pot. And the closer we get to the bottom, the more the population grows and the more amenities people want. Instead of decreasing our demand for raw materials as we get closer to running out, we continue to increase our rate of usage. Which will inevitably cause a crisis.

Interestingly, only certain raw materials have been or will soon be exhausted. Others, you might be surprised to learn, will not. Oil, most famously, is the key resource known to be limited in its reserves. Only a finite amount was formed in the distant past, and once we use that up, it's all gone, forever. Wood, too, has been a limited resource, as those once seemingly limitless forests now appear quite finite indeed, and if we had continued down the path of clear-cutting with unrestrained abandon we would have run into a serious shortage of wood and wood products.

SMART RECYCLING

But other raw materials are not really in short supply at all. Aluminum ore, for example, is incredibly common, constituting 8 percent of the Earth's crust by weight. That's more than we could possibly even visualize consuming anytime in the next several centuries. If that's the case, you may then wonder why we even bother to recycle aluminum cans. If aluminum ore is as common

as dirt, what's the point? Well, this is where things get complicated. While aluminum ore may be absurdly abundant and very
easy to extract, the problem comes with refining it down to pure
aluminum. It turns out that, because of the specific chemical
properties of aluminum, it takes an enormous amount of energy
to extract the pure aluminum from all the other components of
aluminum ore. The only way to do it on any commercial scale is
via electrolysis, which consumes a huge amount of electricity. So
the difficulty in creating raw aluminum comes not from the rarity
or inaccessibility of the ore but from the energy consumption of
the refining process. Recycled aluminum cans, on the other hand,
are already pure aluminum. To recast them as raw aluminum once
again, all you need to do is melt them down—a very simple process, with no electrolysis required. So the environmental benefit
of recycling aluminum actually comes from saving energy—oil,
gas, electricity—and not from saving aluminum per se.

It becomes complicated when you start to calculate the amount
of energy required to do all the steps of recycling at the beginning
of the process. If you were to drive your SUV five miles to the
recycling collection center to drop off a single can, and they loaded
that single can onto a truck and drove to a port, where it was
loaded onto a ship and carted halfway around the world, and then
finally melted down—you'd actually end up using more energy
than you would have if you'd just used raw aluminum ore from
the bauxite mine to begin with. But if you took, say, 20,000
crushed aluminum cans to the recycling center in your SUV, and
they bundled them up with many more and loaded the truck to
bursting, and shipped the cans in bulk to the smelting plant, then
the total energy expenditure *would* be much less than using raw
materials. The difficulty comes in calculating the actual real-world
energy expenditure used for each pound of resulting raw alumi-

num. If recycling is done inefficiently, then it can be a net *loss* in regard to energy consumption, compared with standard mining costs. So one must be very careful not to assume that recycling is always better than using raw materials; sometimes it's not.

Iron, too, is similar to aluminum in regard to its economic and environmental costs. The Earth has no shortage of iron ore—in fact, by weight, our planet is 35 percent iron. Nor is it particularly difficult to extract. The expense comes in shipping it back and forth around the globe, from where it is extracted to where it is processed to where it is used. If iron recycling is done efficiently, it can reduce the amount of energy expended to produce raw iron again. But if done inefficiently, it doesn't really benefit the environment much at all. In fact, it can even be detrimental. The same principle applies to recycling glass bottles, since the raw material for glass (sand) is essentially limitless.

As an illustrative example on a micro scale: A friend of ours, an avid recycler, took a two-week vacation to Nicaragua. While traveling, every time he finished drinking from a bottle or can, or reading a newspaper or brochure, he asked where the recycling bin was. Well, it turns out Nicaragua is not quite as devoted to recycling as is the United States, and our friend's queries were invariably met with blank stares. But he was so used to recycling everything he could that he just couldn't bring himself to throw away his potentially recyclable garbage. So what did he do? He kept it. He decided he had to stay true to his recycling principles and bring everything back home to North America, where he could put it all in the proper recycling bins. So, for his entire trip, he lugged around an ever-growing load of garbage—uh, recyclables—even including "compostables" such as banana peels and melon rinds. He started out with one small backpack and returned with three large bags, bursting with bottles and cans and paper and plastic and rotting organic material. He flew home on a jet airplane, checked his "luggage," somehow made it through customs, and dutifully recycled all those things he had consumed while traveling.

Is he a recycling hero? Or was his well-intentioned adventure ultimately counterproductive? He freely bragged of his exploit, but when questioned about the exact economic impact of what he had done, he became a bit more vague. We pointed out that the jet fuel required to transport the material thousands of miles from Nicaragua to his home probably exceeded the energy savings created by the recycled material in the first place. He brushed aside that possibility. He was too devoted to the concept of recycling to even entertain such a thought.

PROTO-RECYCLING

These days we take recycling for granted. Most large cities (and plenty of small ones) have what is usually called "municipal curbside recycling pickup," whereby residents can place their household recyclables in color-coded bins on the sidewalks in front of their homes, where they are loaded onto trucks by city crews and delivered to centralized collection depots. If you're under thirty you probably have known no other system. But it hasn't always been thus. Prior to the curbside pickup system, if you wanted to recycle, you had to bring the recyclables—glass bottles and aluminum cans only—to a recycling center yourself. And even that system was only made possible due to the little-known but epochal decisions in 1968 by both Reynolds (the aluminum company) and Owens-Illinois (the world's largest glassmaker) to start buying recycled cans and bottles from ordinary people—provided the containers were all gathered and sorted at a local hub to which people had brought them. Prior to 1968, only specialized free-lance scavengers managed the nation's recycling.

Social historian Susan Strasser examines the mostly forgotten story of these freelance proto-recyclers in her book *Waste and Want*: "All over the country, even middle-class people traded rags to peddlers in exchange for tea-kettles or buttons; in cities, rag-men worked the streets, usually buying bones, paper, old iron and bottles as well as rags. These small-time entrepreneurs sold the junk to dealers who marketed it in turn to manufacturers." Actu-ally, during the postwar decades immediately preceding 1968, there was very little recycling of this type going on at an indi-vidual level; the system Strasser describes was thriving during the nineteenth century up through the Great Depression, but after the government-organized scrap-metal drives of World War II, recycling—for a couple of decades at least—was forgotten.

The disappearance of the premodern scavenging class was not necessarily a bad development. Yes, we can glamorize the quaint old days with their frugal customs, but as Strasser points out, a substantial number of these impoverished street scavengers were children, engaged in dangerous child labor and earning only pen-nies per day. Scavengers of the era were eking out a living in the most unsanitary conditions imaginable. We're so used to the an-tiseptic contemporary urban landscape that we forget how abso-lutely revolting cities were before such modern developments as the automobile, biohazard incinerators, the ASPCA, and flush toilets. Scavengers had to cope with horse droppings and pus-soaked hospital bandages and dead rabid dogs and used cloth diapers. And rotten meat and flea-infested cushions and toxic patent medicines and tubercular spittoons. Perhaps it was better to develop a new system after all.

Efficiency measures in some industries also spelled doom for the scavengers of old. For centuries, poor men (and sometimes "swill children") would collect bones from every household along a street, and then sell the bones to middlemen who sold them in large lots to glue factories and fertilizer companies. But the huge industrial meatpacking plants that were supplying steaks for America's tables eventually wised up that they were missing out on a potential profit source; instead of throwing away the bones left over from the meat processing (which had been a common practice), they realized these small-time scavengers were making money by collecting and reselling the very same material. So the meatpacking plants began selling their leftover bones directly to the fertilizer companies, in such massive volume and at such discounted prices that there was no longer any market for the post-consumer bones collected and offered up by the scavengers.

Strasser argues, convincingly, that prior to the mass production of the Industrial Revolution and attendant consumer culture, average people maintained a "stewardship" of household objects. Each item, being individually crafted by a skilled workman, and being comparatively expensive, was cherished, kept, fixed if broken, handed down, and thrown away only if it was utterly beyond repair. When factories began churning out identical household items by the millions, and marketers began encouraging people to dispose of the old (so that they could buy the new), we entered the era of the throwaway society. The scavengers of yesteryear often scavenged the shredded and shattered leftovers of daily use: rags and torn paper and garbage and broken bits. But the throwaway society, despite putting a strain on the environment and causing innumerable sociological changes that we're still trying to come to terms with, actually launched a new golden age for scavengers. Now, instead of having only bones and broken crockery and lumps of coal available to scavenge as in the bad old days, we can go out and discover still-working laptop computers, prom dresses worn only once, stereo speakers, and fiberglass cross-country skis, all tossed out thoughtlessly by uncaring consumers. Strasser decries this throwaway culture and pines for those days when each object was precious and unique; and while we somewhat sympathize with this view, simply out of nostalgia for an era we never personally experienced, on the other hand we revel in this new golden age. Because, as scavengers, we're the ones benefiting from it. In a perfectly efficient world, there'd be nothing to scavenge. And how fun would *that* be? A scavenger's nightmare.

TRASH-HAPPY

"Cognitive dissonance" is a psychological term describing the condition of someone who simultaneously holds two diametrically opposed and mutually contradictory views. Usually it's the first step on the road to the madhouse. And yet, as the authors of this manifesto, we freely admit that we suffer from a sort of philosophical cognitive dissonance that is not so easily resolved. On one hand, we bemoan the thoughtlessness and wastefulness of our modern consumer culture. We curse the corporations that have deluded generations of Americans into assuming that they could get anything they wanted with essentially no effort whatsoever, just by going to a new retail store, picking out their favorites, and "paying" for them by waving around a piece of plastic called a credit card. We reminisce about nonexistent bygone yesterdays, before our consumer culture convinced everyone that they had to lard their lives with shoals of unnecessary *stuff*. We see millions of souls corroded by ease and entitlement and immediate gratification. No one *appreciates* things anymore. When a society removes the need to scrabble or struggle for anything, imagining that by doing so it is giving the gift of prosperity to its populace, what does it do to our collective conscience? Like many other well-intentioned undertakings, it has an unintended side effect: our convenience-themed culture has drained out of us all the ways in which we were once keen, inquisitive, observant, curious, and grateful—personality traits that made us human to begin with.

On the other hand . . . *hallelujah!* The wastefulness and thoughtlessness of all those mainstream consumers only serves to create an endless buffet of treasures for us scavengers. Want to be wasteful? Go right ahead! Because we scavengers will gladly relieve society of its unwanted possessions. If you're foolish enough to buy something at full price and then let us have it for pennies or (better yet) for free, who are we to complain? Furthermore, you've absolved us from feeling any guilt about using up the Earth's resources, because by surviving and thriving on used and unwanted stuff, we're not really making any demands on the Earth at all. In fact, we're saving the Earth from *your* trash. And we get to experience our own lives of abundance and leisure, wallowing in society's endless flotilla of scavengeables. Free stuff, no guilt, life of leisure—we scavengers never had it so good!

So, you may ask, which is it? Do we disapprove of our wasteful consumer culture, or revel in it? Now you understand the meaning of cognitive dissonance, because the answer is "both," even though the two options are mutually exclusive. Does that make us insane? Are we hypocrites? No, and no. The resolution of this moral conundrum is that, as scavengers, we are *realists*. If we had godly powers, certainly we'd protect the Earth and save the environment and make everybody a little more appreciative of life by eliminating the endlessly insatiable consumer culture. But we're honest enough to admit to ourselves that we don't have the power or influence to do that or even put much of a dent in it. So, given that society is the way it is, and there's not much we or anyone else can do about it, we might as well take advantage of the way things are, as opposed to the way things could have been. And that means: Enjoy the bounty of consumer waste! If life gives you lemons, make lemonade. And if life gives you leftovers—scavenge!

SCAVENOMICS = ECONOMICS + PATIENCE

Scavenomics is a bit like cheese-making; the longer something ages, the more valuable it becomes. Take, for example, discarded clothing. People tend to throw away their clothing once it has gone out of style. Everything, however, eventually comes back into style sooner or later, first as kitsch, then as serious fashion, until it is deemed "vintage" or "the classic look." Yet nothing is as embarrassing and has less inherent worth than an article of clothing that just *recently* went out of fashion, when it occupies that no-woman's-land between being currently in mode and being an object of nostalgia. Last year's model is laughable; the model of three decades ago is cool. The same principle applies to many categories of scavengeables. One-week-old garbage is garbage; two-thousand-year-old garbage is an archaeological treasure trove. What this means is that societal waste that seems, under standard economic models, to have literally "gone to waste" by ending up in dumps or trash piles may actually, in the scavenomics model, be *acquiring value* as it ages, like cognac in a cask. That's the beauty of scavenomics: Nothing is beyond redemption. Nothing is garbage. Even its status as "pollution" may be temporary. If we wait long enough, those sealed containers of toxic waste rusting away in a storage facility may one day be recognized as the raw materials for interstellar jet fuel. We just don't know. Yet. What differentiates scavenomics from standard economics? *Patience.*

WHAT IS WORK?

Does scavenging count as "work"? To those among us who are modern-day neo-scavengers, who scavenge for pleasure or simply because we can't control ourselves, the answer is a resounding "No." It's not work, it's *fun*. But what about impoverished Third World dump scourers, or Victorian-era ragpickers, or professional scrap dealers, or any number of other subsistence-level occupations that entail scavenging as a (not always very pleasant) way to make a living? For them, does scavenging count as "work"? While we would now tend to say, "Yes, it's work just like any other job," this inclusive view is a new development. For centuries, scavenging was considered outside the bounds of standard acceptable behavior, occupying a sort of netherworld between having a real job and starving to death. Which was problematic because until fairly recently in Western culture, work, in and of itself, was deemed essential, soul-cleansing, and necessary for human dignity. And scavenging sure as heck didn't qualify.

In 1904, German sociologist Max Weber first enunciated his theory of the "Protestant ethic," now more commonly known as the "Protestant work ethic," or more precisely the "Calvinist work ethic." Weber posited that the attitudes toward labor professed by Jean Calvin and other early Protestant reformers such as Martin Luther were fundamental to the subsequent economic success of nations that adopted Protestantism as a religion. Calvin's theology, which now may seem a little odd to our hedonistic modern brains, was that a man's salvation was not assured by merely engaging in the sacraments and other empty rituals of Catholicism but rather was something given solely by the grace of God. You were either saved or not saved, and there was nothing you could do to change the situation. But how could you *tell* if you were saved or not?

Rather than give in to a passive fatalism, which you might think would be the result of such a theology, Calvin implied that your soul's eventual fate could be ascertained if you appeared to be blessed while you were alive. It was a peculiar self-fulfilling, bootstrapping kind of philosophy that boggles our modern notions of logic, but it allowed for a desperate optimism among the freshly minted Protestants. You may not be able to control whether or not you are saved, but you can control the factors that indicate your state of salvation. If you're "blessed" with success in life, that must indicate God smiles on you, which is a good sign. So do you just sit around and wait for good fortune to come your way? No! You work for it, as if your life—or more accurately your *after*life—depended on it. Furthermore, according to Calvin, accumulated wealth must not be locked away and gloated over but rather put to work and reinvested to increase your business and your blessings.

Before long, the popular interpretation of Calvinist theology became: Worldly success is an indication of spiritual salvation, and hard work brings about worldly success. Thus, work is good for your soul, a sort of cleansing self-mortification that is a substitute for the monastic asceticism of the Catholic Church. The end result of this new worldview, according to Weber, is that when Protestantism became the dominant religion of northern Europe, it brought with it an unprecedented "work ethic" that had never existed before; people for the first time worked more than they needed to and found an almost spiritual satisfaction in it, even after (as eventually happened) the work ethic became a force of its own, divorced from the religion that helped spawn it. And all those people working like never before, combined with scientific and other social changes, led to the emergence of the economic system we now call capitalism. And when every member of society strives desperately to better himself, society as a whole becomes more prosperous, more wealthy, and more successful.

In that preindustrial era, "work" meant being a craftsman or a farmer or a businessman: creating, fashioning, making, being an entrepreneur, building up, up, up. Now, imagine being a scavenger in such a society. Does gathering rags indicate that you are blessed by God? Does foraging just enough discards to survive mark you as successful? Hardly. Scavengers failed to meet the standards of the Calvinist work ethic, and scavenging for the most part was excluded from the category of "work" altogether. Thus developed yet another prejudice against scavenging. If you weren't working, it was very likely you were going straight to Hell. And even though very few people in the modern world *consciously* follow Calvinist precepts today, those precepts remain a hidden cultural motivator, even in the twenty-first century. People (Americans especially) *still* see work as "good for you," see unemployment as misery, regard half-employed or nonemployed scavengers as losers and failures. Because of this lingering bias, economists and just average people have until very recently tended to exclude scavenging-related occupations as relevant components of the economic landscape. As a consequence, faulty models for how the social economy functions—which did not take into account notions such as the full environmental cost of disposing of waste or the financial impact of scavenging—dominated economic theory. The current popularity of "green economics" has rectified that failing to some degree, although green economists focus more on environmental impacts and not on scavenging specifically.

MOTIVATIONS

Scavenging isn't just fun. It's environmentally beneficial. It diminishes the amount of waste, it eliminates the need for overproduction, it helps to decrease the amount of raw materials being extracted from the ecosystem, and so on. We take this for granted: that one of the main motivating factors for scavenging is that it's good for the planet.

At the same time, in this book we are drawing a connection between the scavengers of today and the scavengers of bygone eras. But the motivations for scavenging back then were completely different. A medieval ragpicker or a nineteenth-century scrap-metal collector wouldn't even know what environmentalism *is*; but if you took the time to explain it to them, and then asked if that was the reason they scavenged, they'd look at you as if you were crazy. Saving the wilderness was the last thing on their minds. Humans have always recycled and scavenged, but it is only recently that we do so out of altruistic concern for the planet's well-being. Impoverished people in earlier eras scavenged simply because they were trying to scrape out a living, and collecting things of value from the garbage was the only way they knew how. Colonial-era metalworkers and smiths recycled scrap metal and scavenged discarded household objects for smelting not because they were concerned about the effects of strip mining in Bolivia, but because recycled metals were the least expensive way to get the needed materials for their businesses. It's the "invisible hand" of Adam Smith at work again: people take the path of least resistance when making economic decisions, and sometimes it turns out scavenging is the smartest thing to do even when the only thing you're considering is your own profit.

WHEN YOU SCAVENGE, you absorb other people's pollution like a sponge. Not only do you consume less and thereby decrease your own "economic footprint," when you reuse or recycle other people's trash, you decrease *their* economic footprint as well. Free stuff, and becoming an environmentalist hero to boot—what's not to like?

GETTING SMART ABOUT SCRAP

Waste and garbage and discards all used to be regarded by mainstream culture as a form of impurity, something of *negative* value. Yet as the nineteenth century and then the twentieth progressed, the realization slowly dawned that this was an economic blunder; there *was* value in trash, but we were failing to take advantage of it because of our prejudices. There was an "inefficiency in the market" (to use modern terminology) that nobody was exploiting. Nobody, that is, except for the reviled and despised scavengers of the inner cities. Maybe those rag-and-bone men weren't so stupid after all.

As Carl Zimring details in his history of scrap dealers, *Cash for Your Trash*, it was the iron-related industries that first took advantage of recycling on an industrial scale. Railroads, steel fabricators, the early automotive companies, and other businesses that required a lot of iron paid little attention to the antiscavenging prejudices found in society: they needed a lot of iron, and they wanted it delivered as fast as possible and as cheaply as possible. If they could get a better deal on a ton of scrap metal from a scruffy scavenger than they could from the respectable owner of an iron mine, then so be it. The scrap dealer got the contract.

Part of this seemingly enlightened attitude had to do with the inherently sterilizing nature of steelmaking. Zimring notes that one of the valid phobias concerning salvaged materials in those days was that it could and did serve as a disease vector: rags and old papers and stinky leftovers often hosted vermin and germs that could infect anyone who touched the material. But scrap iron gets melted down by giant furnaces at 2,800 degrees, which need-less to say kills any germs and vermin and removes all impurities. The steel produced from recycled "dirty" scrap iron is just as pure and clean and sterile as the steel produced from raw iron ore.

DUMPING DUMPS

Dumps and landfills used to have a very bad reputation: they smelled nasty, they took up space, they attracted rats and spread disease, they leaked toxic chemicals into the groundwater—all bad no matter how you look at it. Yet things have greatly im-proved. With better management techniques and better presort-ing, landfills (the term "dump" is no longer acceptable; too many negative associations) are now almost eco-friendly. In the new system, already common in Europe and becoming more common every year in the United States, all toxics and most recyclables are barred from entering the landfill and are instead sent to spe-cial processing centers. Now only organic garbage, plant matter, paper, metal (mostly iron and aluminum), glass, some kinds of plastic, fabric, and other types of nontoxic material are allowed into landfills. The contents are constantly turned over and buried by bulldozers, turning the whole place into a gigantic compost pile. Over time, the iron will rust and crumble away; termites will eat and digest the paper; worms will eat and poop out the organic garbage; the fabric will disintegrate; the glass, plastic, and alumi-num will just sit there inertly like artificial rocks; and if you came back in a hundred years, the landfill wouldn't look any different from the surrounding area. Plants will grow and cover everything, and it's likely you would never be able to tell it was a landfill to begin with. A good example is the former city dump in Berkeley, California, which after decades of use was finally filled up and covered over, and is now a lovely waterfront park. So, despite the horror we feel about garbage, it only ends up hurting the environment temporarily. A century or two is just a blink of the eye to Mother Nature; all that garbage will be quickly reabsorbed into the Earth. No matter how diligently we practice recycling, we'll never be able to completely eliminate our society's outflow of garbage. Perhaps we shouldn't get so exercised about its unacceptability, because the new landfill management techniques ensure that in the long run our household garbage won't really damage the environment as much as we currently fear it does. Yes, there are many disreputable old-style dumps still functioning, but little by little they are being shut down and phased out, replaced by new green landfills.

Furthermore, incineration is coming back into style. Not the old kind of incineration that produces noxious columns of toxic black smoke but a new technique called plasma arc gasification, which utilizes ultra-high-energy electrical arcs to not just simply incinerate the trash but render it down to its essential molecular components. The end result of the process is a sterile and non-toxic slag that takes up far less volume than the original waste, and even less space than the ash of traditional incinerators. Even better, the system produces very little air pollution, and depending on the type of waste being "gasified," the plasma arc process will produce outflow gases that can be captured and actually used as fuel. Some of the existing plasma arc plants end up producing more energy than they consume—a net gain. While these futuristic processing plants can be expensive to build, and are still fairly uncommon, they are growing in popularity and may eventually cause us to rethink garbage entirely: no longer a bothersome problem, garbage may one day be viewed as a valuable raw material for generating fuel.

The garbage situation in the Third World, however, mars our

rosy picture. Most dumps there are still inconceivably foul. There is little or no presorting. Toxics contaminate everything. Rats and other disease vectors run rampant. Air pollution and groundwater pollution are unattenuated and unmonitored. Colonies of decidedly unglamorous human scavengers—many of them children— literally live *in* the garbage, barely surviving day to day. All the things that used to be bad about our dumps here in the developed world are *still* bad in the Third World; even worse, the sheer volume of garbage (due to overpopulation) and the variety of potential toxic chemicals have only grown in recent decades. Adding to this nightmare scenario, many of the obsolete electronic components (such as computer monitors) that we so punctiliously "recycle" here in the United States end up getting shipped overseas and deposited in or near these dumps, where specialized scavenger children disassemble them *by hand*, often inhaling mercury fumes and touching other toxics in the process. We have no magic suggestions about how to solve this problem other than to encourage more scavenging here at home to decrease the amount of material that gets outsourced overseas, and to keep pioneering clean landfill and incineration technologies so that Third World nations can eventually emulate our example.

SCAVENGEES

It takes a certain personality trait to enjoy scavenging. Even if you don't mind the potential for social disapproval, even if you're perfectly okay with delayed gratification, and even if you wouldn't mind getting a little dirty in your quest for treasure, you still might not be able to cope with the inherent *disorganization*. Because that's what scavenging essentially is: a conscious reversing of the natural organizational entropy of the human environment, by which everything tends toward messiness. Scavenging entails plucking from that mess the one thing that doesn't deserve to be there. The only real distinction between a standard retail environment and a scavenging environment is that in a standard retail environment you can easily find what you want. In fact it's that ease, that organization, for which you're paying. If you want a pair of green cotton pants with a 32-inch waist, in a regular store you'd just go to the pants department, find its size-32 area, and then look for green cotton pairs. That's it. Takes one minute, very calming. But if you're a scavenger and you want a pair of green cotton pants with a 32-inch waist, you have to wallow through rummage sale after rummage sale, yard sale after yard sale, thrift shop after thrift shop, and so on for an undetermined amount of time in order to eventually (if you're lucky) find what you're looking for. It is this seemingly inconsequential detail that actually scares most people off scavenging. When a rational person looks at a disorganized pile of junk, the last thing they'd want to do is start sorting through the junk and organizing it into piles. Ah, but the scavenger, who must be a little nuts, is excited by the sight of this very same pile, and is overwhelmed by an urge to plunge into the mess—not to wallow in its messiness but to take advantage of the fact that everyone else is scared off.

Because of this, being an active scavenger is not for everyone. Try as we might to convert the world to our way of thinking, we know that a very substantial percentage of people lack the personality trait (some might say personality *flaw*) that would ever make scavenging enjoyable. Yet there are many of you who would like to participate in the whole scavenging movement somehow. And there is a way. Instead of being a scavenger, you can become a "scavengee."

Being a scavengee is easy: your job is to supply the things for scavengers to scavenge. The most obvious example of this is recycling. When you put out your household recycling box for its weekly pickup, or deposit a bottle into a recycling bin, you are admirably participating in the scavenging ethos, but you're not actually doing the scavenging yourself. Someone *else* (in this case the professional municipal recycling crew) is going to scavenge what you've supplied. When you donate clothes to a thrift store, you become a scavengee. Host a garage sale, put out a FREE box, intentionally leave things where others can find them: in each case you are a scavenging supplier. And scavengers love you for it, for without scavengees, there'd be a lot less for scavengers to get. Scavengees are an essential component of the scavenomics cycle, so even if you blanch at the thought of Dumpster diving yourself—heck, you can still join the scavenging revolution.

CHAPTER 5

FOUND STYLE

The Aesthetics of Scavenging

THE LEAN-JAWED MODEL STRIDES OUT ONTO THE catwalk, dark side-parted hair bouncing as his black-jeaned legs slice past a wildly applauding crowd of San Francisco socialites. From his neck to his thighs, a soft poncho flows in alternating woolly bands of charcoal and slate gray, its bottom edge pointy and frayed. Pausing for a split second, he pivots on his shiny black dress shoes and we see that the poncho is pieced together from cut-up old sweaters. Following in his footsteps moments later is a couple in matching formal wear: the peaches-and-cream-skinned brunette in a strapless, skin-tight-bodiced, full-skirted blue gown with flouncy net petticoats visible; her partner in tux and tails. The crowd whinnies in delight. As the pair approach, our suspicions are confirmed: both gown and tux are made from faded old jeans: cut up, reconfigured, reborn.

Other wonders follow: A gauzy cocktail dress constructed

of used panty hose. A conservative suit jacket rendered kooky-cute with a fake-fur collar and fire-engine-red plastic buttons. A black gown made of deconstructed trousers outfitted with a tight leather corset crafted, the announcer tells us, "from an old briefcase." At the subsequent auction, bidding for the corset-gown begins at $1,200.

It's a scavenged-style fashion show. Each of these garments has been made—some by well-established designers—of reconfigured thrift-shop clothes.

A few months later, another crowd—this one mostly young and hipsterish—attended another San Francisco event, the Renegade Craft Fair. In a huge converted waterfront warehouse, thousands of shoppers spent a summer Saturday perusing wares handmade from salvaged goods. At booth after booth, spanning aisle after aisle, each item proved more clever and creative than the last. One booth offered wallets made from cut-up wide neckties. Another sold bowls made from warped vinyl LPs. Another sold skirts sewn from old sheets. To make the blank books he sells under the brand name Recover Your Thoughts, crafter Doug MacNeil explains that he salvages "old books that the library has given up on." After retrieving the books from library discard bins, MacNeil removes their pages and snips off their spines. Between the front and back covers, he sandwiches stacks of blank paper "collected from print shops after they have discarded them"—then attaches spiral bindings. "I take a lot of pride in the fact that I'm able to make a usable product from stuff headed toward the landfill," MacNeil tells shoppers. At another booth, Kim Thomas sells what she calls "B.O.B.s," or "bags out of bags." They're plastic Safeway shopping bags cut up, flattened, sewn together, and processed to make bright, durable, long-lasting purses and totes. "I get the plastic bags from a variety of places: my mom, coworkers, friends, neighbors"—anyone, Thomas explains, whom she sees discarding them. "Also, I have been known to take bags out of the recycle bins at the local Safeway. . . . It's not stealing. It is using them for a better cause." Elsewhere at the fair, other artisans are selling scrap-patchwork stuffed animals, teacup chandeliers, and jewelry made of bottle caps, buttons, plywood scraps, and typewriter keys.

How did we get here?

FOR MOST of human history, a single fashion dictum ruled:
New is best.

It seemed so logical. New clothes ostensibly declare their wearers' wealth and social status.

As such, new clothes fill all who see them with obeisance, even fear.

In a looks-obsessed world, clothes signal personality and loyalty but most of all career and class. For most of human history, dressing below—not at or above—one's status would have been social suicide. To risk being mistreated or losing marital or job opportunities because of outgrown, outdated, worn-out clothes that one *did not have to wear* was unthinkable. Our forebears would have snorted: Who in their right mind would willfully dress as if he or she were poor?

"No woman," warned *Ladies' Home Journal* in 1925, "has a right to look dowdy."

WHEN CASUAL WAS RADICAL

If you could whisk back in time to a late-1940s American city sidewalk, you'd be startled at how dressed up everyone looked.

High heels. Skirts. Hats. Tailored suits. Fur coats. Trousers pressed razor sharp. Even small children: Crinolines. Muffs. Gloves.

And not a T-shirt to be seen. No sweatshirts, stretch pants, sneakers, sandals, leotards. No clothes deliberately slit, no torn-off sleeves, collars, or cuffs. No night wear worn by day. No clashing patterns—well, perhaps on one poor drunk.

To modern eyes, the urban scene of not so long ago would have been barely recognizable: an ocean of uncomfortable, conformist, almost formal fashion. The old dictum "New is best" still held sway uncontested, as did its subtext: Fancy is best. Casual wear and sportswear were not for display on city sidewalks so much as at home, at parties, and at the beach, campsite, and tennis court— if worn at all. My grandmother, who worked in Manhattan department stores, never once wore trousers, although she lived to 1975. More damningly, cheap, comfortable wool or cotton clothes identified their wearers as menial laborers, thus poor; higher-class jobs required more expensive fabrics, higher style.

So when a clique of postwar intellectuals in San Francisco and New York City started wearing cheap, comfortable wool and cotton clothes in public on purpose, America was shocked.

Now we call them the Beats. They were poets, novelists, essayists, artists, scholars, and Ivy League dropouts who became overnight sensations after the 1957 publication of *On the Road*, Jack Kerouac's fictionalized account of his own cross-country saga, aswirl in sex and wine-sparked stream-of-consciousness. Appearing in magazines and on live TV, Kerouac and his friends slouched in frayed and faded sweaters, sweatshirts, T-shirts, chinos, jeans, and checkered cotton shirts such as ranchers or railway men might wear. (T-shirts, developed in England as men's underwear circa 1880, were not yet generally considered acceptable outerwear: footage of soldiers sporting uncovered T-shirts during

World War II had scandalized the public, as did James Dean's T-shirt scenes in *Rebel Without a Cause*.) Beat gear was the direct opposite of what that era's previous discontents wore: zoot-suiters and jazz-scene hipsters dressed with rococo extravagance. That shabby clothes displayed the state of cerebral spontaneity that Kerouac—who coined the term—called "beat" is clear from frequent references in *On the Road* itself. A hitchhiker rejecting the American dream, we read, "wore a beat sweater and baggy pants." The book's subversively sexy antihero, Dean Moriarty, wore "greasy wino pants with a frayed fur-lined jacket and beat shoes that flap." As portrayed by Kerouac and his followers, such clothes declared their wearers rough but deep, at home with bricklayers and Rimbaud. Like most intellectuals, the Beats wanted it both ways. They displayed this by inventing shabby chic. And what better, "beater" way to buy it than secondhand?

In *The Dharma Bums*, his 1958 follow-up to *On the Road*, Kerouac lauds a Berkeley grad student/Buddhist/anarchist/mountaineer named Japhy Ryder, who was based on the real-life poet Gary Snyder. Japhy, we learn, was irresistible to pretty girls. Seeking him out at all hours, they climbed onto him for wild sex in exotic positions. In public. In the mid–twentieth century. And *he wore used clothes.*

"Japhy's clothes were all old hand-me-downs," Kerouac wrote, "bought secondhand with a bemused and happy expression in Goodwill and Salvation Army stores: wool socks darned, colored undershirts, jeans, workshirts, moccasin shoes, and a few turtleneck sweaters that he wore one on top of the other in the cold."

In one scene, Kerouac and Japhy go to working-class Oakland with their friend Alvah—based on the real-life poet Allen Ginsberg—"to some Goodwill stores and Salvation Army stores to buy various flannel shirts (at fifty cents a crack) and undershirts. We were all hung-up on colored undershirts . . . foraging with bemused countenances among all kinds of dusty old bins filled with the washed and mended shirts of all the old bums in the Skid Row universe. . . . I bought a nice little canvas jacket with zipper for ninety cents."

That was a boast.

And it changed everything.

Thrift- and surplus-store work clothes became cool—less for women than men, who thronged to dress like Kerouac & Company in flannel shirts and colored undershirts and frayed jackets and baggy pants.

It's hard to grasp now how outrageous that was then.

U SED CLOTHES had always, invariably, reeked of shame. They were plain proof of poverty. Only by dire necessity would one wear what others had junked, because it was dirty, damaged, or out of style. Through much of history, even *selling* used clothes was stigmatized. During the Renaissance in France and Italy, it was one of very few jobs permitted to the much-hated Jews. In Israel Zangwill's novel *Dreamers of the Ghetto*, we watch "sore-eyed wretches trundling their flat carts of secondhand goods" around the slums of sixteenth-century Venice, where these miserable "forced vendors of secondhand wares" were known as *strazzaroli*. Centuries later, poor people bought moth-eaten frock coats and greatcoats and other outdated clothes at seedy eighteenth- and nineteenth-century London markets such as Petticoat Lane— which was named for the goods sold there. The reason that museums today display almost exclusively the clothing of the middle class and rich is that the poor wore their clothing until it fell apart. Wearing used clothes was a source of shame. "They call me Secondhand Rose," sang Fanny Brice in the 1922 chart top-per. "Things I'm wearing someone wore before," the singer la-ments, citing a series of used items in her wardrobe. "It's no wonder that I feel abused."

Even though used clothes began to acquire panache in the post-Kerouac era, the old stigma did not disappear overnight, lingering well into the 1960s. The same shame and horror were still very much alive in Dickey Lee's 1962 song "Patches," about "my darling of old Shantytown" who drowned herself because others mocked her much-repaired hand-me-downs. A little beg-gar wearing torn, ill-fitting clothes—encountered en route to a recording studio—inspired the Four Seasons' 1964 hit "Rag Doll," which sighs: "Such a pretty face should be dressed in lace." And not, we are meant to understand, secondhand lace.

In their 1968 classic "Love Child," the Supremes invoke a woman scarred for life by that horrible long-ago day when "I started school in a worn, torn dress that somebody threw out."

FOUND ART

Antiques were another matter entirely. Considered precious be-cause of their original face value, used art and fine crafts and jewelry have almost always been objects of pride. Priced as such, they do not count as scavenged style. But a new aesthetic began to emerge in the twentieth century. Striving to elevate scavenged objects into fine art, in 1917 the artist Marcel Duchamp bought an ordinary urinal from a New York City ironworks, titled it "Fountain," and presented it at an art show. Yes, he had bought the urinal new rather than scavenging it, but to art-world sophis-ticates it looked like something from a junkyard. That was

Duchamp's point. He presented a whole series of other used-looking, quotidian items—a snow shovel, a dog comb, a bicycle wheel—which he altered slightly and called "readymades." These confirmed his membership in the spontaneous, absurdist, anti-art Dada movement, a precursor to the irony and nihilism that shades much of the arts today. Duchamp wrote that he hoped his ready-mades would inspire "a reaction of *visual* indifference with at the same time a total absence of good or bad taste . . . in fact a complete anaesthesia." The glory of a readymade, Duchamp wrote, "is its lack of uniqueness." Gloating, he declared the bike wheel "absolutely devoid of aesthetic pleasure."

This idea of mass-produced everyday objects as elements of style sparked widespread disgust back then. It has since become a keystone of scavenged style—and of *all* style. In 2004, a panel of British art-world elites voted "Fountain" the most influential artwork of the twentieth century.

But when the Beats burst onto the scene, secondhand goods were still considered mostly junk. Mainstream society back then would have scorned the little table made of old orange crates at which Japhy Ryder sat studying Zen poems.

RISE OF THE HIPPIES

Kerouac was no left-winger. Flag burning enraged him. He supported the Vietnam War. Kerouac died in 1969, too soon to fully understand how the scavenged style he had popularized almost single-handedly would be passed down, with slight variations, from one radical subculture—the Beats—to the next—the hippies. He wouldn't have liked that. Because he disagreed violently with hippie politics.

With its Buddhist and skid-row sympathies, Beat culture idolized the underdog.

But so did Karl Marx and his philosophical acolytes.

As history has proven, scavenged style and socialist-tinged youth rebellion ended up being a perfect fit.

IT IS ALWAYS the goal of subcultures to shock the squares. At the time it feels fun, significant, world-changing, and original, as long as your friends are doing it, too. For the Beats, merely wearing used clothes was a revelation and a revolution. Ten years later, used clothes as such were not enough. Hippies acquired them for cheap—or free—then raised the bar by beading and fringing and cropping and tie-dying not just work clothes but Victorian, Edwardian, ethnic, and formal wear, mixing eras and styles to turn their bodies into art and circuses, political debates and Rorschach tests. For the first time in history, looking au courant meant looking totally individualistic: wearing not what everyone else was wearing but what *no one else was wearing*—at least not in the same way, in the same combinations.

"For my parents' generation, wearing a fur coat was a status symbol," remembers Colleen Redman, a writer who grew up near Boston, in her blog. "For us in 1969, it was counterculture chic, but only if it wasn't new. It had to be ragged with wear and tear to be really cool." Nor could it be worn "straight," in its original context, but rather with a miniskirt or faded jeans—barefoot, or with sandals or boots. In an interview about hippie fashion for the *Sunday Mirror*, Welsh homemaker Ann Fowler, who conveniently transposed the letters of her last name to call herself "Flower" in 1967, "used to love this long, flowing skirt—I bought it in an Indian shop." She wore it with a jacket that "was actually a pyjama top. My great-uncle was in the Merchant Navy and he'd brought it back from China."

"The yellow embroidered dress over the yellow trousers were typical hippie attire," muses British clothing-shop owner Jan Price, in the same interview. "I used to spend hours sewing beads, fringes and sequins on to my clothes. I even put shells and bits of wood on my dresses, but it sounds mad now, doesn't it? I used to dress like that to go [to] pubs reading my poetry. It was all protest stuff at the time—we all thought we were saving the world."

Hippies haunted thrift shops and "free stores"—incomparable, anarchic emporiums where at absolutely no cost, customers took as much as they wanted whenever they wanted from an ever-shifting array of donations and discards. In the 1968 film *I Love You, Alice B. Toklas*, Peter Sellers portrays Harold Fine, a strait-laced lawyer who accompanies his hippie brother Herbie to a Los Angeles free store.

"What is this," Harold asks, gazing around him at the racks and boxes overflowing with gowns, neckties, and top hats. "A hippie supermarket?"

"Yeah." Herbie grins. "See the clothes? . . . Those clothes are free."

"They're old," Harold protests.

Herbie points to a customer, a shabby-looking man: "They're new to him."

"What you're trying to say," Harold declares, "is it's a form of, uh, communism."

"No, no, no, no," Herbie demurs. "It's, like, love."

He picks up a book.

"Hey, Harold," says Herbie. "This is a groovy book."

It is the quotations of Mao Zedong.

Later in the film, Harold himself becomes a hippie. A huge Ho Chi Minh poster hangs on the wall of his pad.

In 1967, a *New Yorker* reporter toured the East Tenth Street free store and found it "crowded with Negro and Puerto Rican children, old women speaking Middle European dialects, barefoot runaways with glazed eyes, stumbling winos, and gaily ornamented hippie couples, all picking through boxes full of used shoes or fingering racks of soiled clothing." One young woman, the reporter observed, "wears a Mexican riding blouse of white muslin unbuttoned down the front to reveal a purple T-shirt with a silk-screened portrait of 'the Zig-Zag man.' . . . On her head she wears a 'Rigoletto' hat of dark-red velvet, with dyed ostrich plumes, which she found in a carton of contributions from a theatrical-costume shop." The first free stores were in San Francisco, operated by a radical cooperative called the Diggers. The most famous Digger free store was Trip Without a Ticket, on Cole Street in the famous Haight-Ashbury district.

FOUNDED IN 1966, the Diggers named themselves after a group of seventeenth-century British back-to-the-landers often credited as the first communists. Although many hippies were primitivist Luddites, the twentieth-century Diggers viewed technology as a wondrous force that would liberate humankind from having to work. In the Diggers' vision of a utopian future, someday—sooner rather than later, they hoped—machines would do all the jobs that had always kept men and women trapped in countless offices and stores and factories. Thus freed of drudgery, the people of the world would lounge and love in never-ending peace. Scavenged style, the Diggers believed, was one step on that path.

Their plan was to excite the masses about the idea of everything becoming free. Published in the August 1968 issue of Paul Krassner's magazine *The Realist*, a Digger manifesto vows "to convey the flavor and feeling-tone of a revolutionary community" and "to spread [our] word: free." Digger protocol, which largely became hippie protocol, was to precede all possible nouns with the adjective "free." Free love. Free clinics.

Free clothes.

Clothes should neither be bought nor sold nor hoarded, because "the Diggers are hip to property," the manifesto read, indicating that they disdained the notion of possession. "Everything is free, do your own thing. Human beings are the means of exchange. Food, machines, clothing . . . are simply there. Stuff. A perfect dispenser would be an open Automat on the street. Locks are time-consuming. . . . So a store of goods or clinic or restaurant that is free becomes a social art form." Free stores, the manifesto asserts, are also "ticketless theater," where "life-actors" assemble scavenged-style outfits with which to convert squares—whom the Diggers dubbed Establishment "wardens."

"Theater is territory," the manifesto proclaims. Seeing outrageous outfits, wardens must "react to life-actors on liberated ground."

It's no surprise that the Diggers drew so much upon dramaturgy. The group's founding members had belonged to the San Francisco Mime Troupe, which performed (and still performs) skits—mainly Marxist and Maoist-flavored, mocking American traditions—for free, creating a form of scavenged entertainment. The troupe's founder, R. G. Davis, defines his inspiration thus: "Western society is rotten in general, capitalist society in the main, and US society in the particular." The Diggers expanded on this. Their 1968 manifesto declares:

"Fire helmets, riding pants, shower curtains, surgical gowns and World War I Army boots are parts for costumes. Nightsticks, sample cases, water pipes, toy guns and weather balloons are taken for props. When materials are free, imagination becomes currency for spirit."

And for revolution. "Guerrilla theater," the manifesto avows, "creates a cast of freed beings."

THAT IDEA appeals to many scavengers today, as do the Diggers' dreams of no one having to work and everything being free. But lethal flaws lurk in those promises. Sooner or later (actually, sooner), all the free stuff would run out. If no one worked, who would produce more stuff? And if some putative unnamed workers *were* to do the creating, how would those who made stuff be paid, since no one could make a profit *giving away* their products? *Oh, but there's no need for wages or payment, you say, because there's nothing to buy; everything's free! Remember?* Well, then, if everything's free, what motivation would anyone have to volunteer in a grim factory churning out the necessities of comfortable living while everyone else is frolicking and having orgies outside the factory gates? With no incentive to work, no one *would* work, and nothing new would ever get made, and within a very short time we'd all be scrabbling for the few remaining fragments of unshredded clothing. An entire economy consisting of nothing but scavenging as the only mode of behavior would quickly disintegrate. Scavengers survive by being a minority among huge numbers of eager standard consumers. We use what is in effect their effluence. Their consumption and wastefulness sustain us. Digger optimism excludes the reality of what would happen in a world where everything was free: the vicious and the strong would steal it all. To some extent, this happened in the free stores. Reflecting on the New York store, Marty Jezer remembers that it "became a focus for trouble," that his famous fellow activist Abbie Hoffman was regularly "called in to deal with the street toughs who would storm through the store intimidating and sometimes beating up the hippies."

Female customers, Jezer reports, were dragged out of the store and gang-raped. Incidents of vandalism included a metal trash can hurled through the store's window. Nonviolent but predatory nonetheless, professional secondhand dealers made off with merchandise in bulk—free stores could not prohibit this—and sold it. "In perhaps the most pointless robbery in the history of the United States," observes the Haight-Ashbury historian Charles Perry, "the Diggers' Trip Without a Ticket free store was burglarized."

THUS FAR, scavenged style had continually proclaimed a self-contradictory set of beliefs. Marx, Mao, Ho, and Kerouac championed the worker. But the Beats were not really workers, except as a lark; they were actually intellectuals. The Diggers were inspired by communists and radicals. Their 1968 manifesto offers a list of idols that includes Fidel Castro, Huey Newton, Malcolm X, "Mad Bomber" George Metesky, and—among other artists, poets, and activists—Gary Snyder, the real-life version of Japhy Ryder, and Neal Cassady, who was the real-life model for *On the Road*'s Dean Moriarty. For both the Beats and the hippies, scavenged style signified freedom. Yet Mao, Ho, and Castro were repressive dictators. While American and European hippies lounged in jeans and cowboy boots, on the far side of the world young Chinese people were being tortured and killed for even *owning* Western clothes. In the communist societies the Diggers idealized, total conformity of clothing, behavior, and thought was ruthlessly enforced.

As uniforms for ideologies, scavenged style had as a result become tainted with hypocrisy.

SWINGING LONDON

But even while its wearers vowed to overthrow the Western world, scavenged style was becoming a commodity. Capitalism is very, very sneaky that way. At any point in history, whatever the young, pretty, and famous wear cannot help but be co-opted. Janis Joplin, observed one journalist, "ambles onstage wearing the spoils of a raid on a thrift shop." In 1967, at the murderous apex of China's Cultural Revolution, a *Time* reporter noted "Carnaby Street regulars" sporting Red Guard uniforms while strolling through London's trendy boutique district.

"With youth," the *Time* reporter gushed, "the 'antique look' this spring is in. Students in Paris and London have been ransacking secondhand stores for old uniforms dating back to the Crimean and Franco-Prussian wars." Their American counterparts sought secondhand mobster gear such as old silk "palm tree–studded ties and double-breasted pinstripe jackets. At Dartmouth, the particular 'drinking uni' (for uniform) at the moment is . . . a Red Baron Flying Ace helmet, complete with ear flaps and shrapnel holes. At Harvard, the grapevine passes the word around within hours" whenever the local Goodwill store "gets in any old taxi-driver hats or brown-and-white shoes."

In London, scavenged style soared from the depths of dowdiness to high fashion within a few short years. In flea markets that had previously been haunted only by the poor, early-'60s Mods and musicians and young elites sought creative alternatives to the dour conformity that had dominated British fashion since before the war—and the scarcity that had persisted both during and since. One such seeker was Jane Ormsby-Gore, a onetime girlfriend of Mick Jagger—and the possible subject of his song "Lady

Jane." Raised in a titled Welsh family that hobnobbed with royalty, Ormsby-Gore hated what she calls the "fluffy and puffy"
dresses that aristocratic young women of her era were expected to
wear. Interviewed for a fashion history exhibition at the Victoria
& Albert Museum, Ormsby-Gore recalled recently how an early-
1960s trip to America whetted her appetite for scavenged style.
In a nation transformed by the Beats, she bought blue jeans, then
transformed them into hip-huggers by snipping off the waist-
bands and ripping out and resewing the leg seams. To make them
look older—that is, more scavenged—she washed each pair four
times before wearing it. Back in London, "I started buying lots of
secondhand clothes and mixing and matching and cutting,"
Ormsby-Gore remembers. "Then, I think because of my amusing
way of dressing, I was asked to work for *Vogue* . . . selecting things,
finding things that I thought were interesting." Even so, she
wasn't allowed to wear trousers at *Vogue*'s London office.

Ormsby-Gore treasured her scavenged goods: "I remember
finding a shoe buckle with huge great emeralds," albeit fake ones,
at a flea market. "I loved that sort of thing . . . suddenly to have
flashy jewels which you wore with your jeans, which now everybody wears all the time." But scavenging components at widespread shops and markets was time-consuming. At that point,
"nobody actually gathered [used] things together and made them
into a shop." Her husband opened just such a shop, Hung on You,
on King's Road in trendy Chelsea. It swiftly became a landmark
in what the media liked to call "swinging London."

I Was Lord Kitchener's Valet was another such landmark. It
was "this secondhand shop that sold strange things at the top end
of the Portobello Road," remembers Robert Orbach, who began
as a customer—and a Mod—but later became the store's long-
time manager. Acquiring inventory was easy. "It was only fifty or

so years from Victorian times, when we had an empire. We used to buy fur coats by the bale." In 1964, IWLKV stocked "racks of tunics; there were boas, those old fox stoles, secondhand fur coats, pith helmets, Victorian dresses, bits of Victorian furniture, general junk, some good and some bad. Some people liked wearing secondhand clothes" in 1964, Orbach explains, but not many. Not yet. So "at first it wasn't that busy." But soon, "you had all these rebels without causes, and all of a sudden at one moment in time everything came together."

And it came together in secondhand stores, as rock stars discovered IWLKV.

"Eric Clapton was the first one to buy a military jacket, early in 1966, when Cream's first album came out," Orbach remembers. Others quickly followed suit.

"I'm sitting there one morning and in walked John Lennon, Mick Jagger, and Cynthia Lennon. And I didn't know whether I was hallucinating . . . but it was real. And Mick Jagger bought a red Grenadier guardsman drummer's jacket, probably for about £4 or £5." Jagger wore the high-collared, figure-hugging coat while singing "Paint It Black" on the TV music show *Ready Steady Go!* in 1966.

"The next morning," Orbach remembers, "there was a line of about 100 people" outside IWLKV. "We sold everything in the shop by lunchtime."

By 1967, IWLKV was a chain, with two spin-off stores thriving on King's Road and just off Carnaby Street. Other famous customers included the Who and Jimi Hendrix. Hendrix was often photographed in his cherished Royal Hussars regiment jacket, adorned with ropes and tassels. The artist Sir Peter Blake claims that an IWLKV window display provided his inspiration for the *Sgt. Peppers Lonely Hearts Club Band* album cover.

THE BIRTH OF VINTAGE

Within a few years, scavenged style had pretty much ceased star-tling anyone. But for most of the '60s, "New is best" still domi-nated the straight, middle-class, middle-aged world, as manifested in an ever-expanding number of shopping malls. By the early '70s a fashion transformation began to take place that would have astounded Patches, the darling of old Shantytown. An aesthetic began to arise in which scavenged goods, *as* scavenged goods, were admired by unprecedented numbers of middle- and upper-class consumers. But there could never be enough truly scavenged clothing to satisfy the demands of the majority of all consumers; scavenging by its nature must necessarily be a fringe activity of the few, since it siphons off the discards of the mainstream. So, at some crucial unnamed moment in the early '70s, mainstream de-signers sensed the swelling demand for scavenged style and began intentionally manufacturing brand-new clothes to *look* like they were old and scavenged, even though they had just come from the factory. And nothing's been the same since. The cycle of co-option had started. From that moment onward, whenever a new scavenged style appeared, it was rapidly copied and marketed by new-stuff designers. The name of a new jeans brand that became trendy in the early '70s—Faded Glory—reveals all.

By the '70s, comfortable work wear and casual wear were ac-ceptable almost everywhere. It was the era of the leisure suit. And urban streets had changed irrevocably, aswirl in T-shirts, shorts, jeans, sneakers, and sandals.

Augmenting this casual revolution, World War II–era and postwar sportswear was flooding secondhand stores. Cast off by middle-aged and older owners, these were the clothes once worn at home, at backyard barbecues and cocktail parties: Hawaiian shirts, loud jackets and ties, and halter tops. Their hues and patterns exuded a sense of victory: tropical bright, bold black-and-white, shot through with silver, copper, gold. Flowers and fruit, sunbursts and abstract blobs, alluding to travel and outer space. Their buttons were often novelties, too: coconut shell, seashell, bamboo, faux or real foreign coins. While the Beats and the hippies scavenged unwanted clothing from the Victorian era through the 1930s, the new generation of fashionistas began to scavenge the discarded clothing of postwar America—since that's what was available.

It stood in sharp contrast to what hung on the standard retail racks back then: a lot of solid beige. Brown. Orange. Yellow. At the mall one day I asked my best friend's mother to name the strange amorphous color of some sack dresses we saw. She held up a sleeve and admired it.

"Olive drab," she said. The fact of being young at a time when drab was considered pretty made my blood run cold.

That was the decade when the human touch visibly vanished from culture and commerce. Those were the growth years not just of malls and corporate conformity but of synthetic fabric, synthesized music, processed food. Even "earth tones," as olive drab and its ilk were then called, came from synthetic dyes, though they were designed to emulate the color palette of old and ethnic clothing. Stadium rock transformed us into livestock. Disco was a factory of polyester- and spandex-clad clones. Amid all that newly manufactured ugliness, secondhand sportswear in those days was becoming popular again, but refracted through a '70s lens: Watergate, recession, post-Vietnam PTSD, pot-smoke stupor, cocaine haze. The type of postwar scavenged style popular in the '70s bespoke nostalgia for a bygone era whose naïveté and hope and joy seemed gone forever. Not that one could admit this *during* the '70s. It would have made one seem as if one cared, and for many of us in the '70s it was imperative never to care.

By then, scavenged naïveté and hope and joy meant irony and apathy. By then, scavenged style was sexy not because it signified solidarity with something serious but because it did not. It was the look of the sardonic, thus the smart.

And it went by a new name: *vintage.*

Far removed from its role as proletarian guise, and further removed from its role as shameful *strazzaroli* wares, vintage meant venerable. Thus it meant *valuable.* This euphemism lent second-hand gear a dignified identity, not new but nice and clean and socially approved. It could even sound haughty, spoken down the nose. *This top? It's vinnntage.*

So while it could still be bought for supercheap at thrift shops and other such venues, that colorful postwar clothing was increasingly corraled into a new genus of retail operation: the midprice vintage boutique. A new breed of middle-class teenager spent long afternoons combing the racks at stores such as Aardvark's Odd Ark, with several outlets all over California. Bought at bottom dollar and often in bulk from sources lower down the used-goods chain, its used merchandise was cleaned and organized for easy shopping, just as at mall stores: jackets here, khaki pants there, sundresses over there. These boutiques were more plebeian than their swinging-London ancestors, with all chaos removed. Becoming easier and easier to acquire at ever higher prices, vintage-style scavenged style as it emerged in the mid-'70s was arguably more *style* than *scavenged.* Winning a Best Picture Oscar, Woody Allen's 1977 film *Annie Hall* was about a modern woman who loved to wear vintage ties, vests, bowler hats, men's shirts, and baggy '30s-style trousers. In actuality, the costumes worn by star Diane Keaton hadn't come off the thrift-shop rack but were designed by Ralph Lauren. The look swept America, influencing the fashion industry at every level, spurring a boom in imitation vintage wear. Reproduction Hawaiian shirts and halter tops and baggy '30s-style trousers filled racks at Macy's, Sears, and Kmart. One could look as if one was wearing scavenged style without ever scavenging a thing.

PUNK FASHION

And into this ambience, screaming *Fuck this* and *Fuck that*, erupted punk. With it came new versions of scavenged style. In New York City, one of punk's two primary birthplaces, the skinny-jeaned, leather-jacketed, slightly unisex punk look was a natural, if snide, heroin-inflected update of street-tough cool. In London, its other birthplace, the look merged labor (via Dr. Martens work boots) with sadomasochism (via bondage-fetish accessories such as studs, chains, and zippers) and a dash of fascism.

An ex–art student turned fashion designer, Malcolm McLaren operated a King's Road boutique called Let It Rock. "I sold the ruins of pop culture . . . ancient jackets in leather, velvet, and tweed resembling clothes worn by such dead stars as Eddie Cochran, Gene Vincent, and the Shangri-Las," McLaren later recounted. But, he said, "I was bored with it all. Bored with the same surrogate suburban teddy boys that drifted in from God knows where. Bored with the hippies and refugees of Chelsea's swing-ing '60s looking for charity and kindness. Bored with the demands of the BBC wardrobe department and their dreadful revivalist TV shows." Sick of '70s-style scavenged style, McLaren "was lost in dead tissue."

On a business trip to New York in 1974, McLaren met the New York Dolls, an edgy band whose look, sound, and persona were poised between glam and proto-punk. Its members wore flamboyant secondhand gear, some of which was drag: feather boas, stretch pants, schoolgirls' uniforms. The Dolls "were so, so bad, they were brilliant," McLaren recalls now. He became their manager. Back in London, "I decided to change my shop and call it Sex, a place for liberated teens." There he sold bondage-fetish gear inspired by the Dolls. And there he met John Lydon, a skinny young customer who wore a scavenged-style T-shirt; over the silk-screened words PINK FLOYD, Lydon had scrawled I HATE. McLaren was forming a new band, the Sex Pistols. He signed up Lydon as its lead singer, christening him with a new punk name: Johnny Rotten.

Such names were part of punk-style scavenged style, which, unlike its predecessors, focused not on beautifying salvaged goods but on flaunting their filthiness and ugliness, even making them worse. Classic punk tactics entailed plucking clothes (preferably skintight and preferably black) from Dumpsters and not washing them but slashing them and writing or spitting on them, or worse, then wearing them. Punks told the world they felt like trash: the disaffected discards of an industrial wasteland, furious and bored. Especially in the early days, some punks wore Hefty bags with slits cut for their heads and arms. ("We're the flowers in your dustbin," sang the Sex Pistols.) Even at its less extreme, punk fashion involved altering used clothes, attaching metal fixtures that suggested violence. "That black school blazer I renovated late last night has turned out fantastic!! Bolts, bath chain, razor blade, safety pins etc on the widened lapels look great," wrote Adrian Fox, then a sixteen-year-old London fanzine editor, in his 1977 diary. Norm Fasey, rhythm guitarist for the band the Violators, remembers "wearing homemade gear. Painted army-surplus jacket with stenciled Clash-type writing. Old school trousers made into drainpipes"—skinny straight-leg pants—"and a shirt with 'Fuck Off' painted on the front." Simone Stenfors, whose punk name was Mrs. Suicide, remembers: "I used to go into my dad's wardrobe and steal everything I could off him. I used to nick his big shirts and ties and wear them with footless tights, stilettos and Lurex socks. I used to wear miniskirts, lots of makeup, jackets with rips, safety pins and chains."

Punk music, too, was scavenged style. Band members were chosen and stars made based purely on attitude and will, on what McLaren calls "a fundamental belief in the strength and purity of the amateur over the slickness of the professional." It was a jubilantly raw DIY world. Punk posters and fanzines were written or typed at home, photocopied at the local shop, and circulated locally for free. In one now famous 1976 issue, the British fanzine *Sideburns* published diagrams for three basic guitar chords with the caption: "this is a chord / this is another / this is a third / now form a band." Trained or talented or not, you played whatever instrument was nearby. Throughout his entire career as the bassist for the Sex Pistols, it was common knowledge that Sid Vicious barely knew how to play the bass. This did not stop the band from attaining icon status. While some punk musicians were true virtuosos, many succeeded for other reasons entirely.

Nor was punk's secondhand style nostalgic. Punks loathed pretty much everything that had ever happened, everywhere; their secondhand style was spiked with violence, despair, in-your-face ugliness. The hippie in *I Love You, Alice B. Toklas* describes free clothes as "like love." Punk-style scavenged style was like hate. It howled, *Look at me!* and simultaneously, *Fucker, how dare you look at me?*

It was a consummately consumerist era. So even something as seemingly unmarketable as an antishopping antifashion was commodified as well. And once again the mainstream embraced a scavenged style without having to do any actual icky scavenging.

Punk became a marketing gimmick. Clothes were manufactured to look torn, stained, bleach-splattered, and safety-pinned. This made life easier for those who didn't want to take the trouble of creating punk-style scavenged style themselves. Unlike its predecessors, punk-style scavenged style was difficult, its elements requiring preparation: damage, yes, but it was work. Beat gear and hippie gear and vintage gear had been easy to find, ready-to-wear. Tie-dying and beading were optional. Wannabe punks, known (and despised) as poseurs, bought their gear brand-new, prepunkified. (They still do, as distressed clothing is still in style. At one of many such garment factories in China's Guangdong Province, thousands of workers systematically scrub, spray, and rip jeans to produce 10,000 distressed-look pairs a day—for export to the West, of course.)

Punk-style scavenged style expressed boredom and hate, but *whose* boredom and hate? Punk was all over the ideological map, so the same torn Dumpster shirt and schoolgirl skirt meant vastly different things depending on who wore them. As punk grew, it split into substrata, so that some punks—like Richard Hell—were nihilists. And some—like Joe Strummer—were socialists. Others were anarchists. Others were racist skinheads, others antiracist skinheads. The Sex Pistols called themselves anarchists but were nihilists as well. Their lyrics were self-contradictory.

We're the future.

There's no future.

Punk couldn't make up its mind—maybe because it was too bored—whether its scavenged style was meant to invoke oppressed laborers or genocidal storm troopers. The punks' only unifying ideology was to hate the free-and-easy hippies who preceded them and also to hate the artificial disco scene that symbolized unoriginality. When Malcolm McLaren managed the New York Dolls in 1975, he decided "to make them look not like girls, but worse, like Communist dolls. Red, patent-leather Communist dolls. I had a fondness for all that Chinese stuff." Retro costumes were duly assembled, and a stage set. "Red was the colour and I thought it needed to be their colour." At one famous concert, a hammer-and-sickle banner hung onstage. McLaren handed out copies of "a manifesto of sorts that declared the politics of boredom: 'Better red than dead.' The Dolls came onstage soaked in a ray of red light." Singer David Johansen "waved Chairman Mao's Little Red Book. Everyone drank red-coloured cocktails and sat on red upholstered chairs." Of course, this ironic political posturing was all just shock theater for the masses; McLaren was the consummate capitalist. A few years later, Sid Vicious was widely photographed wearing swastika T-shirts. Siouxsie Sioux, lead singer of Siouxsie and the Banshees, sported a Nazi armband. Nazi regalia, both genuine and reproduction, was ubiquitous in punk-style scavenged style. Some punks said they sported Nazi gear not because they admired Hitler but to annoy their elders who still felt emotional about the war. (In other words: to shock the squares.) In his diary, Adrian Fox wrote about wearing an "old silver and green-striped boarding school tie (with a swastika earring)," but lamented a few days later, "I lost my Nazi earring . . . a fucking loss at that!"

Punk was politically amorphous, but the mood its scavenged style conveyed—rage, resistance, depression, destruction—has continued to dominate youth culture ever since. From grunge to goth to death-metal and beyond, wherever you see ripped, ragged, bleach-splashed, and/or purposedly wrong-sized clothes, they are punk legacies. When Nirvana front man Kurt Cobain committed suicide in 1994, after a short stratospheric career, the *New York Times* obituary began: "Dressed in thrift-shop plaid shirts and

torn jeans, a fashion soon copied by designers around the world,
Mr. Cobain . . . raged against the material and synthetic trappings
of pop music." Whatever the genre, such clothes are now meta-
phors for not fitting in.

CONTEMPORARY SCAV STYLE

But punk and grunge are just two streams of scavenged style
among zillions. Since the Beats, scavenged style has expanded and
diffused throughout the world so thoroughly that every individual
scavenger today has his or her own personal version—from the
highly specialized to the rough uncut kind, in which one literally
wears or decorates with whatever one finds. Early '80s underground zine *Nancy's Magazine* once ran a satirical article taking
the concept to the extreme, advocating that its readers wear
costumes consisting of the least likely scavenged items imaginable, such as a dress made out of typewriters, hula hoops, and
Saran Wrap. Out there in the standard-consumer world, new is
still best. But ex-hippies and ex-punks and ex-grunge fans now
hold powerful positions in the fashion, entertainment, media, and
merchandising industries. Consciously or not, they give scavenged
style more and more exposure. Hosted by breezy blond craft designer Wendy Russell and aired via the Home and Garden Television (HGTV) cable network, the Canadian-made series *She's
Crafty* features such found-art projects as turning old books into
birdhouses and old telephones into clocks. An entire cable network, the DIY Network, reaches 50 million American homes
with shows about do-it-yourself activities such as scrapbooking,
jewelry-making, and home repair, many of which use found or
thrifted elements. The "craftster" movement, which also often

employs found and scavenged goods, mushroomed in the first decade of the twenty-first century. Boston-area computer programmer Leah Kramer started Craftster.org in 2003 as a way to display her DIY experiments such as coffee-machine lamps and Popsicle-stick purses. The site rapidly expanded to more than 100,000 members. By 2008, the site was gaining thousands of new users every month. Hundreds of craftsters sell their wares via Etsy.com, an enormously popular website launched in 2005. Etsy oversees millions of dollars in sales every month—with an ever-shifting itinerary ranging from car-key charm bracelets to Ramen-noodle-packet slippers. A new genre of craftster handbooks emerged with the new millennium, packed with ideas for making CD racks out of cut-up Scrabble boards and wallets out of tennis racquet covers. Aimed at young adults, these books make a point of insisting that the projects and the spirit they invoke are a whole new thing, a *cool* new thing, not at all the same thing as when Aunt Hilda used to make toilet-roll covers by crocheting dresses onto tacky plastic dolls. The authors are postpunk, pierced, often posturing as fierce. In *Bizarre Bazaar: Not Your Granny's Crafts*, for example, Greg Der Ananian details making marbles into fridge magnets and fast-food wrappers into quilts.

When cutting-edge New York City fashion designer Miguel Adrover included an inside-out used Burberry raincoat in his autumn 1999 show, he made the cover of *Women's Wear Daily*. Adrover has also made a dress from discarded mattress fabric and a skirt from a dismembered Louis Vuitton purse. Jonathan "J.J." Hudson, founder of the trendy London fashion-design outfit Noki House of Sustainability, attracted celebrity patrons with his series of salvaged cheap '80s T-shirts, their printed logo designs faded and fissured, to which he added ballpoint-pen graffiti and handmade "moth holes." Chinese artist Yin Xiuzhen uses sewn-together "found clothing" to cover her steel-framed sculptures. One of Yin's installations was composed of two model airplanes, each seven yards long, sheathed in rugby shirts, underwear, T-shirts, and floral blouses. Mainstream travel guides list secondhand shops side by side with ordinary retail stores. In Rome, the Travel Channel recommends Fuoriserie and Marcolino.

So today we are as likely to see professors sporting patched army-surplus khaki pants as we are pastors wearing vintage ties, hipsters hanging found art in their flats, supermodels wearing strategically tattered haute couture, and teenage rock stars wearing earth-tone polyester thrift-shop shirts. Scavenged style today is several generations deep. Many young people have no idea that the looks they assemble retail, at full price, are actually imitation scavenged style; they realize neither that the pretorn, prefaded, appliquéd clothes preprinted with scrawled messages are meant to look old nor that the looks originated decades back. Retailers sell newly manufactured replicas of items that might have hung in a Diggers free store forty years ago—such as $54.95 patchwork pants at the Hippie Shop in Fairfield, New Jersey, whose promo blurb reads: "Bellbottoms became extremely fashionable in the late 60's and continued to be popular through most of the 70's. Using various patches of baby corduroy and cotton, some with embroidered designs and some with floral patterns, we've taken this old design and added a new twist." The twist, not really new, is a drawstring waist.

Generations deep, scavenged style references itself like a hall of mirrors. Wearing not your own era's version of scavenged style but some earlier era's carries urgent implications. The sexually inquisitive young heroine of Haruki Murakami's 1999 novel *Sputnik Sweetheart* "wanted to be like a character in a Kerouac novel—wild, cool, dissolute. She'd stand around . . . staring vacantly at the sky through her black plastic-frame Dizzy Gillespie glasses," the narrator tells us, "which she wore despite her twenty-twenty vision. She was invariably decked out in an oversize herringbone coat from a secondhand store and a pair of rough work boots." She dresses this way hoping observers will understand what it means.

Fashion magazines, design houses, and clothing manufacturers no longer have the patience to wait around for a new scavenged style to catch on and take root all by itself, the way hippie style and punk style and grunge style did before being co-opted. Those were the naïve old days. Now there is keen competition to see who can identify and copy the latest emerging minitrend before anyone else does. To that end, many of these very serious adult companies hire young-looking style scouts who hang around high schools and music clubs, scanning the crowds for that one creative trendsetting hipster kid who's ahead of the curve. These trendsetters are called first-adopters. The scouts will even interview *un*hip kids, asking them, *Who does everyone copy at this school? Who's the coolest?* Once the campus fashion royalty has been identified, their every quirk is carefully noted. If one designated cool girl, on a whim, decides one day to use an old coffee can as a purse, two months later there'll be coffee cans lined up in the purse sections of department stores across America.

USED CLOTHING BECOMES FASHIONABLE AROUND THE WORLD

Scavenged style is even disrupting the new-clothing industry. At the dawn of the new millennium, Poland was experiencing a used-clothes boom, with still-fashionable wearables imported in bulk from the West being sold at some 16,000 stores nationwide.

In 2002, the Polish government issued a ban on the sale of imported secondhand clothing. The ban's supporters said their intent was to "civilize the clothing market" and to save the ailing Polish textile industry, to which used clothes presented "unfair competition." Stylists, actors, models, and other celebrities gathered to protest the ban. British *Vogue* reports that they "donned their trendiest [secondhand] clothes and carried pink balloons to try and persuade their government that scouring secondhand shops for unusual clothing was a right they were keen to maintain." Even after the ban took effect, some wholesale importers remained in business. The tagline of Gdansk-based 4Fit company is "Second Hand Clothes in big bags from Great Britain." A photo gallery at the website of the Bydgoszcz-based Dortex company proudly displays long-haul trucks (bearing the firm's logo, three female silhouettes clad in formal gown, business suit, and punk-style torn skirt) barreling down snowy roads, then unloading reefs of clothing into a warehouse.

Other countries, including Bolivia, Indonesia, and the Philippines, have passed similar bans. Ostensibly the goal is to protect local jobs and industries and to guard against purported health risks linked to used clothes. (Yeast infections and foot-and-mouth disease are the leading culprits, if you must know.) Opponents of importation to developing nations call the practice "clothes dumping." The arrival of goods in bulk from overseas, they argue, is a "quick fix" option that deters the rise of new industries.

How does clothes dumping work? As much as 75 percent of the clothing donated to charities in Western countries ends up in the Third World. Far more is donated in Britain, northern Europe, and North America than could ever fit into existing Western thrift shops or even be absorbed into domestic free-clothing programs for the poor—so a substantial proportion of the goods dropped into Western donation boxes is collected, with permission from the charities, by for-profit wholesalers. In exchange for this privilege, the wholesalers donate predetermined amounts of money to the charities. Then they sort the goods, sell the highest-quality items to Western vintage boutiques, and ship the bulk in fifty-kilogram compressed bales to developing nations. There they are resold again and again as dealer after dealer takes portions farther and farther into the hinterlands: "At times," mused a reporter from *The Guardian*, watching women fight over used shirts in a Zambian marketplace, "the whole of Africa seems to be an immense open-air bazaar of Western hand-me-downs."

Secondhand-clothing exports to developing nations from the United States alone more than doubled between 1990 and 1997, according to a United Nations report. In poor but appearance-conscious cultures, style *is* scavenged style. Anthropologist and material-culture expert Karen Tranberg Hansen argues that shoppers in countries such as Zambia, where she did her research, don't simply accept whatever secondhand items come their way but select their purchases very carefully and then often alter them to create countless unique effects. Their version of scavenged style is "about being in the world," Hansen asserts. "It's about abundance and choice." In Zambia, where as many as 75 percent of the clothes bought are not bought new (and where, just to give you a sense of perspective, teachers earn the equivalent of one dollar a day), secondhand clothes are known as *salaula*, a Bemba verb meaning "to rummage through a pile." In his 1988 song "Salaula," the Zambian singer Teddy Chilambe exults over "this bale you have given us . . . that is where *salaula* is found." In Uganda, Kenya, Nigeria, and Tanzania, secondhand clothes are called *mitumba*, Swahili for "bale." In Haiti, to which a steady stream of secondhand goods has been exported from the United States since the 1960s, it is called *pepe*. There, as in Africa, secondhand clothes are often altered to personalize and update them. In *Secondhand (Pepe)*, a 2007 documentary about the Haitian used-goods scene, a woman shows how she has cut and sewn a pale blue blouse to make its long sleeves short, then added darts and a tailored waist for a sleeker fit. "Pepe," another woman explains, "has allowed people to adopt the look that is on television."

For poor Haitians and Africans, as for the Poles protesting their government's ban, the point of wearing secondhand clothes is not that they are secondhand. In a perfect world, these shoppers would rather wear new clothes: New is best. But in their countries, new clothes—either locally made or imported—are either scarce or expensive or both. So scavenged style is the closest they can get to looking as if they are wearing new clothes. Unlike many Western versions of scavenged style, developing-nations-style scavenged style is not an attempt to look destitute.

"These clothes make people's dreams come true," a *mitumba* vendor in Nigeria told a *Los Angeles Times* reporter. "Everyone wears them. . . . When they put them on, you can't tell rich from poor."

GREEN STYLE

The idea that so much donated clothing is actually sold for a profit is shocking. But consider it a form of recycling. At least it keeps tons of material out of landfills and keeps that material from being incinerated into toxic fumes. Discarded clothes that *aren't* donated and sold but that simply stay in the trash and enlarge the world's dumps are in one sense more worrisome. Research by the resource-efficiency consultancy Oakdene Hollins reveals that of the 1.7 million tons of clothing discarded annually in the UK, only 26 percent is diverted for recycling or reuse: that is, donated rather than simply thrown in the trash. The same report reveals that 1 million tons of clothing are discarded every year in Japan, with a minuscule 12 percent being recycled or repurposed as secondhand clothes and industrial wipes. By definition, scavenged style is recycled style. Which makes it the official uniform of the green and DIY movements.

Doing-it-yourself has been around forever. It's how the wheel was invented. The Industrial Revolution aimed to make it obsolete. Thus DIY was a nostrum for hippies and punks. Assembling and crafting their own outfits, decor, posters, and magazines from trash and scraps, they raised the image of DIY from the realm of geeks and rubes and grandparents to the apex of urban chic: something done to save cash but also to make a point. To the hippies, that point was community, creativity, and spontaneity. To the punks, it was looking like trash. In the twenty-first century, it means reducing waste.

If recycling is a new era's mission and passion, then scavenged style is its best option. It shrinks the growth of major polluters such as mills, dyeing plants, and factories while also shrinking landfills and reducing the use of waste-burning factories. This is scavenged style as not just a look but proof that the wearer has a heart. This is scavenged style as sexiness with a conscience.

This is scavenged style as save-the-Earth style.

And its time has clearly come. "Recycled paper bags collaged on a bare wall provide a textured look similar to antique leather or stucco," promises Ecologue.com, one of thousands of green-decorating websites. Torn-out Yellow Pages are another alternative that "solves the vexing question of what to do with outdated phone books. The phone numbers in the listings and the graphics in the advertisements give the wall a fun, eye-catching edge, and the muted yellows and grays are surprisingly sophisticated." The spirit pervades not just hipsterish venues but also established, formerly conservative ones as well. Venerable *Sunset* magazine, which for more than a hundred years has offered home-and-garden tips to middle-class West Coast residents, devoted not just one feature in its March 2008 issue to scavenged style but several, including "Salvage with Style: Turn Secondhand Finds into Decorating Gold." Its photo spread showed thrift-shop housewares arrayed around an attractive flat.

The Western world's thirst for save-the-Earth style has spurred new industries in developing nations, where handicrafts fashioned from salvaged materials such as bottle caps, nails, wire, and food wrappers are now made and sold in increasing numbers for export. Collected at landfills and industrial dumping areas, the "junk" is reconfigured into traditional artifacts: cloth dolls, for instance, might now be made of and dressed in scrap cloth, or wind chimes formerly made of shell might now be made of jar lids. But in many cases the handicrafts, while made of old "junk," are brand-new in inspiration and design. Often under the guidance of Western wholesalers or aid organizations, people who never made crafts before are now assembling items specifically for sale in the West. In Mexico and the Philippines, discarded juice boxes are made into picture frames and tote bags. The Filipinas Fair Trade Venture Group teaches destitute Manila trash-dump dwellers to roll strips of torn magazine pages into tight beads, then assemble huge numbers of these to make vases. They also make bowls from rolled-and-coiled newspaper. In Vietnam, soda cans are cut and bent to make intricate model cars, ships, planes, and helicopters: to trumpet their scavenged-style status, the cans' colors and company logos remain intact. The ships' sails and the cars' hoods say COKE and FANTA.

HIGH FASHION *À LA* SCAVENGING

San Francisco's annual thrift-shop fashion show, Discarded to Divine, was founded in 2005 by the St. Vincent de Paul Society. Every year, internationally renowned designers are invited to participate—dismembering and reconfiguring merchandise from the society's thrift shops into haute couture. Proceeds from the show benefit the city's homeless. For DTD 2008, designer Jessica McClintock repurposed yards and yards of salvaged white netting into a floor-length wedding gown that she titled "Un Visage Romantique." The venue for the 2008 show's preview gala was the venerable de Young Museum. There, under the same grand roof that covers priceless paintings by American masters including John Singer Sargent and Wayne Thiebaud, the city's wealthy and well connected cast approving gazes on haute couture made from what was once considered junk. Other scavenged-style fashion shows are becoming increasingly visible annual events, from New Zealand's Trash to Fashion to the Recycled Fashion Show in Phnom Penh, Cambodia. At the 2007 Recycled Fashion Show, one resplendent Cambodian model wore a sleeveless sheath made of thin, shiny pink plastic, dotted with flamboyant flowers made of cut-up paper plates. Another wore a black trash-bag gown with a wide-brimmed hat made of crushed soda cans. Hundreds of thrift shops around the United States, such as Karen's Kit'n Kaboodle in Spring Hill, Florida, and Treasure City in Austin, Texas, host their own runway shows.

"Lindsay Lohan sizzles in racy photo shoot . . . wearing SECOND-HAND clothes," the UK's *Daily Mail* blared in June 2008. Posed in a miniskirt and oversized suit jacket held slightly open to expose bare breasts underneath, Lohan "showed she was proud to wear second-hand clothing as part of a campaign for ethical fashion . . . wearing vintage clothes in a bid to encourage people to swap their unwanted threads." The star was promoting an upcoming London clothing swap sponsored by Visa. "She had no trouble making the recycled clothing look like [it] had just come off the shelf of a designer store," and the reporter gushed that Lohan "looked stunning in the second-hand attire."

In March 2007, under the headline "Thrift Like a Celebrity," an article in *Glamour* magazine explained: "Ever since Kate Moss stepped out in a gorgeous canary yellow prom dress she found in a secondhand store in 2003, the fashion world has been going vintage-crazy." While stars once sported next season's designer clothes, "now the easiest way to score style points is to announce your outfit once belonged to someone else. A long time ago." Moss "is often seen flicking through the rails of Rellik . . . in Notting Hill. Several of her iconic pieces, like those Westwood pirate boots, have been lucky finds in this cooler-than-thou secondhand shop. Kate also caused a stir when she spent an hour trying on clothes and shoes in Cornucopia in Pimlico, known for its 'Miss Haversham–style' Victoriana." Among other reports on the strategies of other celebrities, we read: "Victoria Beckham has been an advocate of vintage for years now. . . . When Posh was spotted picking up a neat little black dress in a branch of [British charity thrift-shop chain] Oxfam last year, we knew that charity shop chic had hit the mainstream . . . bravo, Mrs B!"

Interviewed during Paris fashion week, Dame Helen Mirren told the *Daily Express*, "I love secondhand shops."

Scavenged style shocks no one anymore.

FASHION: EDITED AND UNEDITED

How scavenged is your style?

Even when it comprises actual not-purchased-new elements, scavenged style can still be classified into degrees: we call one end of the spectrum raw/unedited/unfiltered scavenged style and the other end of the spectrum cooked/edited/filtered scavenged style. The cooked/edited/filtered version is the kind that requires little effort to get. This is the kind assembled at Rellik, Aardvark, eBay, and other such venues whose wares were scavenged—just not by you. Others back there along the retail cycle found, sorted, selected, sanitized, and presented the not-new but now only vestigially scavenged wares amid a this-is-cool-so-*buy-it* ambience. A basic rule of thumb is that the more you pay for scavenged style, the more cooked it is. You pay for others to scavenge your "scavenged" style.

The raw/unedited/unfiltered kind is made up of what you find yourself: *whatever* you find, on your own, in situ. Raw/unedited/unfiltered scavenged style is literally random. No example does it justice because no two examples are even slightly alike, but here is one from life. One day we found a thick, Frisbee-sized plastic moon. It had a smiling face—and batteries inside, and a motion detector, so that walking past it made it sing: *When the moon hits your eye like a big pizza pie, that's amore!* Bringing it home, we hung it in the foyer. It became the foyer's focal point. It sang two dozen times a day. This drove us mad, but being committed to raw/unedited/unfiltered scavenged style, we were compelled to hang it, *had* to keep it, just as monks are compelled to stay celibate and Girl Scouts have to help old folks across the street. Raw/unedited/unfiltered scavenged style is not so much a style as an antistyle, by virtue of which it is actually a hyperstyle. (Fortunately, the moon broke after a couple months.)

Cooked/edited/filtered scavenged style lets you dress or decorate around a theme, a "look" to call your own. Romantic, say, or all stripes or all nautical. It proclaims: *Lookee! This is my identity.* It wants attention. It wants to be clocked as oh-so-clever, oh-so-carefully selected scavenged style.

Raw/unedited/unfiltered scavenged style never lets you pick themes. It telegraphs no single shallow, readable motif about you—*He loves Elvis,* say, or *She's so '70s*—by which you might be patronized, infantilized, marginalized. Instead it shouts only *I am a scavenger.* By virtue of which a spectator might surmise just about anything about you, anytime. Given the hour, given the day—as raw/unedited/unfiltered scavenged style is ever protean—a spectator might scorn you as a hobo. Or worship you as a prince. The trick of raw/unedited/unfiltered scavenged style is that the spectator might never even realize your style is scavenged at all.

Cooked/edited/filtered scavenged style retains many classic scavenged-style virtues. History (it's not new). Mystery (who wore this before, and where and when and with what?). And even cooked/edited/filtered scavenged style is more original, diverse, DIY, eco-friendly, and potentially intriguing than mainstream mass-produced fashion that's purchased new. But cooked/edited/filtered scavenged style omits what is arguably the main virtue of scavenging itself:

Discovery.

And raw/unedited/unfiltered scavenged style is all about discovery.

It is a walk into the wild, a circumstance of total luck and total trust. You absolutely, literally take what comes. That is the vow you take and the promise you keep. It is an adventure, a covenant, a game, whether you end up in Gucci or overalls, whether you end up on a Bauhaus armchair or a faux-leopard-skin pouf. You do not choose your style. It chooses you. As such, you are not predictable, identifiable, or narrow. Raw/unedited/unfiltered scavenged style will not permit you to be "read" or classified.

NONETHELESS, any scavenged style *is* scavenged. And as such, the possibilities are endless. Wearing it or decorating with it renders you and your environment an ever-shifting babel. An archive. An artwork. A recycling center. A puzzle. A university. A sanctuary. A refuge of rescued nows and thens. Raw or cooked, acrylic or Bauhaus, diamonds or Pyrex, scavenged style is the last refuge of the true individualist.

•

CHAPTER 6

FINDING YOURSELF

What Kind of Scavenger Are You?

THE PAINTING SHOWS A SCRAGGLY-BEARDED MAN of indeterminate age, slouching bow-legged in baggy, torn trousers and a grimy, too-big, V-necked peasant shirt. Old shoes immersed in the furled, street-grazing hems of those pants curl slightly at the toes. One of the man's hands holds a filthy-looking stick—for walking? Poking? Stirring trash? The other clasps what looks like a burlap sack, the dun of dirt itself, slung over one sloped shoulder. Perched on his tilted head, a black derby hat is too small, its former elegance ironic given the jutting cheekbones in a face that looks both starved and resigned to its fate, given the scattered litter at the man's feet: onion skins, eggshells, torn paper, broken bottle. That arched nose: Is he meant to look Jewish?

Édouard Manet's painting *The Ragpicker* captured the image that—in 1865, when he began the four-year task of creating it—came to mind when ordinary people heard the word "scavenger." The raddled man in the picture looks lonely, dirty, hungry, poor.

If an artist were to paint a scavenger today, what would the person in that painting look like?

Maybe lonely, dirty, hungry, poor.

Or—

It could just as likely be a fresh-scrubbed student outfitting her first apartment with flea-market furniture. Or it could be a CEO metal-detecting at a pricey beach resort. Or it might be a soccer mom comparison-shopping for uniforms online. Or it could be coworkers at a clothing swap. Two neighbors haggling over blue Ikea dishes at a yard sale. A child finding a coin on the street. Lecture attendees nibbling wine and cheese at a reception afterward. Crowds at a department-store sale. Library patrons. A family stocking up at a discount outlet. A fashion designer transforming recycled burlap into haute couture. It might be your Aunt Ella clipping coupons. A muscular Dumpster diver. An Academy Award–winning actress who adores thrift shops.

All of these and more are scavengers.

All of these and more are getting stuff for cheap or free.

As stereotypes shatter and as prejudices fade, getting stuff for cheap or free is no longer a shameful last resort to be performed only in desperation or in secret. So many of us scavenge now, in so many ways we might not even recognize as scavenging. As thrift shops multiply, as freecycling networks spread, as reuse becomes cool, we have become a demographic.

And a *diverse* demographic. Each of us chooses our favorite form—or forms—of scavenging. Each carves out a new scavenger identity. As stereotypes shatter and as prejudices fade, we should honor them all.

What kind are you?

THIS CHAPTER is really nothing more than a roll call of scavenger identities. A list of professions, handed to the newcomer: Which do you choose? What do you want to be? What *are* you right now?

Most of the people reading this book probably already fit into one of these identities. More than one, because they're not mutually exclusive. If you're one kind of scavenger, if you have the temperament to scavenge, then you probably do it a dozen different ways. Or perhaps this chapter will awaken you to the fact that you've been a scavenger all along, without even realizing it. For reference, on the facing page is a handy list of the many different types of scavenger identities. Each is detailed below. Feel free to add your own.

RETAIL SCAVENGERS

Scavenging doesn't have to mean finding stuff for free. Nor does it have to happen outside the store environment, or for that matter outside the traditional money-for-goods dynamic. Scavenging means getting stuff in any legal way besides brand-new/full price. Sometimes that still means buying it—just not for much.

Yard Saler (and Garage Saler and Rummage Saler)

In many ways, especially for beginners, yard sales are the ideal, one-size-fits-all scavenging venue. Typically held on the lawns or driveways of private homes, usually on Saturdays and Sundays, weather permitting, these leisurely, neighborly confabs are a handy way for households to declutter by selling unwanted possessions, usually very cheaply. Having determined the locations of a given

RETAIL SCAVENGERS

Yard Saler

Flea Marketer

Estate-Sale Devotee

Thrift Shopper

Bargain Hunter

Discount-Outlet Shopper

Coupon Clipper

URBAN SCAVENGERS

Dumpster Diver

FREE-Box Forager

Free Marketer

Finder

Aftermather

Urban Gleaner

Library Lizard

Recycling Poacher

SOCIAL SCAVENGERS

Freecycler

Freegan

Clothing Swapper

Free-Sample Forager

No-Cost Gardener

SPECIALTY SCAVENGERS

Metal Detector

Beachcomber

Treasure Hunter

Prospector

Professional Archaeologist

Amateur Archaeologist

Rural Gleaner

Found-Object Artist

day's sales by examining the local classified ads, Yard Salers plot a route, based either on geography or on which sales look most promising, and depending on whether they are traveling by car, bike, or foot. Because yard-sale inventories can be quite sparse—especially at sales swept clean by the dreaded first-arrival "early birds"—most Yard Salers visit as many yard sales as possible in a single day. All this stopping-and-starting makes yard-saling labor-intensive. Yet for Yard Salers, it's almost all about the process. (*Almost.*) Traveling from sale to sale feels retro, as if one were a frigate captain docking at remote islands, or a medieval sojourner following the Silk Road to haggle at caravansaries. Even if a whole day yields no purchases—or, say, just a wind-up plastic sushi that cost fifty cents—at least it was spent mostly outdoors.

Yard sales feel soothingly familiar. The sellers are just folks, not professional hawkers who must make a living off whatever they can weasel out of you. Yard-sale hosts just want their stuff gone. They don't want to haul it back into their houses at day's end. They don't even want to haul it into their cars and drive it to Goodwill. They're highly motivated to sell and, as the day progresses, to sell cheap. Yard Salers love the interchange and the true stories sellers tell about their merchandise:

This was my favorite hat.

We bought this on our honeymoon.

My mom made this for Justin.

Yard sales first started occurring in the United States during the 1960s. Economic hard times in 1969 and the 1973–74 recession, when many middle-class Americans lost their jobs and needed cheap shopping alternatives, made yard sales increasingly popular. The vintage-clothing fad that began in the '70s further popularized yard sales, which according to one scholar's estimate generated nearly a billion dollars in 1981 alone. Even then, researchers believed that more than half the American population attended yard sales, at least once in a while. So many of today's Yard Salers are second-generation.

Sometimes, yard-sale hosts don't know the real value of what they're selling. They vastly underprice, say, the box of vintage comics they found in the attic that was left behind by a former tenant. They're charging five bucks for the $2,000 Maruman Majesty Prestigio golf clubs their dad gave them before he died. Thus arises a question of ethics. If a seller ignorantly underprices something valuable, do you tell her? Granted, sellers should know *beforehand* what their merchandise is worth. You don't see professional auto dealers charging twenty bucks for 1967 Mustangs. If you reeeeeeally like the seller and can live without the item, sure. Speak up. But only if.

A garage sale is, theoretically, a sale in which someone empties out the contents of his or her garage, but in practice there is no functional difference among a yard sale, a garage sale, and a tag sale—just different regional terminology for the same thing.

A rummage sale is like a hundred yard sales all rolled into one—*without* the negotiable prices and the chitchat. Most are benefits for schools, houses of worship, and the like, so their prepriced (but almost always very low-priced) merchandise is the accumulated ex-possessions of dozens of families, arranged on long tables, usually indoors. Like yard sales, rummage sales are personal, but not *inter*-personal. The donors are not standing around telling you the histories of their stuff. Before leaving, you pay a cashier by the door.

Flea Marketer (and Swap Meeter)

Flea marketing is a blood sport.

The shy need not apply.

Yard sales and rummage sales are mellow. Flea markets are walks on the wild side. While yard and rummage sales are casual affairs hosted by plain folks, a flea market is a large and long-established group of stalls, each stall independently operated by a professional vendor. To say that prices are negotiable is an understatement. Flea-market protocol around the world is that sellers set ridiculously high starting prices only fools would pay. Flea Marketers must argue, parry, feign disinterest, start to walk away as bargaining ensues. Flea Marketers have nerves of steel.

Flea Marketers are patient. They can do math in their heads. They are actors. Debaters. They can dish it out *and* take it.

Flea markets are often historic landmarks, occupying the same plaza or street for centuries.

Flea markets are also notorious sources of fake antiques, fake artifacts, fake name-brand products, and stolen goods, sold by professional hawkers who will gladly lie, humiliate, and berate you in public if it helps them make a sale. Meanwhile, pickpockets frequently ply the aisles.

Flea Marketers endure.

Flea Marketers are even further disadvantaged at markets in foreign countries because local etiquette, different from place to place, applies. For instance, aggressive haggling is considered rude at Tokyo's sprawling Togo Shrine, where savvy Flea Marketers smile and ask politely, *"Makete kudasai?"* (Best price?)

Flea-market-style transactions—semiprivate, semiformal, and often semilegal; one-on-one—are an ancient tradition. In the Middle East, where the preferred term is *bazaar* (from the Middle Persian for "place of prices") or *souk* (from the Arabic for "market"), flea markets thrived during the Middle Ages. The term "flea market," used not only in America but also in France and Italy, is said to date to the seventeenth century and alludes to vermin-infested sellers and wares. Paris's Les Puces de Saint-Ouen market, renowned as the world's largest, with more than 100,000 shoppers on fair-weather weekends, was founded in 1885. For at least a century before that, scavengers known as *crocheteurs* ("pickers") and as *pêcheurs de lune* ("fishermen of the moon") had roamed the city by night, salvaging items from trash heaps that they resold wherever possible. Dubbed *bric-à-brac*, these found goods became a local specialty. In his 1848 novel *Cousin Pons*, Honoré de Balzac exults over his beautiful city, "in which all the curios in the world manage to come together." Persecuted by civic authorities, the *pêcheurs* banded together and began selling their wares side by side at the Porte de Clignancourt. Cairo's Khan el-Khalili, named for the Emir Djaharks el-Khalili, who built it in 1382, was originally a caravansary for traveling traders. Now the size of an entire village, it is immensely popular with tourists. That's why el-Khalili was the target of a terrorist bomb in April 2005. Of the eighteen shoppers wounded, eight were American and European tourists. In all the world, only one flea market is known to be open every day: Brussels's Marché Place du Jeu de Balle, founded in 1873 and featuring more than four hundred stalls.

Many veteran scavengers avoid flea markets and their cousins, swap meets, because of the hucksterism, hassle, crowds, and whiff of crime. Flea Marketers, however, boldly rush into the fray. They know to set limits beforehand: Bring not one cent more than you are willing to spend. Remain calm no matter what. Promise yourself not to get *very* upset if what you buy turns out later to be broken, fake, or stolen.

Caveat emptor.

Estate-Sale Devotee

Estate sales *look* like yard sales. They are held in and around private homes, and the merchandise constitutes the contents of those homes. But while yard-sale hosts are still alive, the former owners of estate-sale merchandise are usually dead—or have recently been compelled, usually by age or illness, to leave their homes abruptly, never to return. To liquidate their belongings, private estate-sale companies are hired by the next of kin to assess and price each item in the house, then manage the sales, usually for a percentage of the profits. The resulting atmosphere feels oddly cold and stilted, not to mention ghoulish. All the accumulated souvenirs of an extinguished life are manhandled by strangers in the very rooms where these items were used and loved for years and years. The clown-shaped cookie jar. The papier-mâché dachshund. The rack of spoons, each from a different Welsh town. The foot-shaped ashtray that says *We got a kick out of West Palm Beach.* It breaks your heart. Yes, merchandise in thrift shops, antique shops, and flea markets often belonged to individuals now dead. But buying it at some remove affords those dead some dignity. Walking their halls, poking into their dresser drawers and bathrooms—in which towels and shampoo and the sea-urchin night-light are price-tagged, too—one feels like a marauder or a burglar. As if that weren't bad enough, estate-sale prices usually aren't negotiable.

Estate-Sale Devotees are mission-focused. Many are serious collectors banking on the likelihood that merchandise formerly owned by someone now old or dead includes valuable vintage stuff and antiques. Such items cost more at estate sales than at yard sales, but much less than they would at antique shops. Entering a house where a sale is being held, Estate-Sale Devotees chuck any vestige of sentimentality and stride directly to the dolls or sheet music or whatever they collect. No fuss, no muss, no chat.

Mission accomplished.

Thrift Shopper

Thrift Shoppers are the most common type of scavengers. With some 10,000 thrift shops peppering the United States—the Salvation Army alone runs 1,300—there are probably more Thrift Shoppers in this country than Yard Salers, Flea Marketers, and Estate Salers combined. This is because thrift shops are the gateway-scavenging venue, the one that most closely resembles a standard consumer store. Because they *are* stores, operating in a reassuringly storelike way with racks, clerks, cash registers, and mild ambient music, *yet are astoundingly cheaper than regular stores*, thrift shops feel like an alternate universe, like how stores would be if we made up the prices.

Thrift shopping is easy, which is not to say that Thrift Shoppers are lazy. Thrift Shoppers are connoisseurs. They know the hours and locations of all nearby shops. They know which shops are best for buying what. They rank the stores by choosing staple items such as white T-shirts and coffee mugs and going from thrift shop to thrift shop, comparing prices in each.

Upon crossing thrift-shop thresholds, Thrift Shoppers often feel a distinct physical sensation: a flutter that is both anticipation and relief. Thrift shops are low-pressure, low-key, and so well stocked—a deft Thrift Shopper could compile a whole wardrobe in a single visit—that, for Thrift Shoppers, they are havens, welcome wagons, outposts, safe houses, shrines, meditation centers, and spas all rolled into one. Yank a Thrift Shopper away from his home turf, fly him anywhere else in the world, and plunk him down in an unfamiliar town. He's lost, disoriented, panicked—until he sees a thrift shop.

Ahhh.

Most of the United States' 10,000 thrift shops are operated by charities. Although Goodwill is secular, its founder was a Methodist minister, Edgar J. Helms, who created a Boston-area employment agency and job-training program in 1902 for disabled and otherwise disadvantaged adults. His slogan was "Not charity, but a chance." The Salvation Army was founded in 1878 by street preacher William Booth and his wife, Catherine, whose mission was to save the souls of Victorian London's homeless and destitute—including its pickpockets and prostitutes. Organized in a military format, with William Booth addressed as its general, other ministers addressed as lieutenants and commanders, and its gospel-preaching converts seen as soldiers, the organization spread to the United States in 1883, where it was endorsed by President Grover Cleveland. Still an active ministry, the Salvation Army calls its retail outlets Family Stores rather than thrift stores. Other charities also began opening secondhand shops during the 1920s. Using the motto "We turn your trash into cash," the Junior League's Washington, D.C., store divided $16,000 in proceeds among four children's-aid institutions in 1931—and they're still at it today around the country. The Quaker-affiliated Oxfam famine-relief nonprofit opened its first "charity shop" in Oxford in 1948; with more than seven hundred shops, Oxfam is now the UK's largest such operation.

Bargain Hunter

Some scavengers buy brand-new stuff—without paying full price. Hunting for bargains is a form of scavenging, whether you do it at a yard sale or online or in a superstore. Researching deals and sales at mainstream stores, then going to investigate, takes time and effort. Bargain Hunters comparison-shop, seeking cheap brands, discontinued lines, generics, economy-size packages, rebates, discounts and sales, and alternative retail options such as catalogs and websites. Bargain Hunters are shocked at how few standard consumers bother to do this. Bargain Hunters are not necessarily poor. In fact, arguably most aren't—having achieved financial security by bargain hunting. After a while, bargain hunting becomes instinctual. Equations glimmer in Bargain Hunters' heads. In the scavenging world, few moments feel more like victory than finding a good deal. So simple. Yet so hard.

Bargain Hunters ridicule brand loyalty. And apparently they're right. Blind taste tests often reveal that generic store brands taste as good to customers as name brands. One such test, commissioned in 2005 by the Private Label Manufacturers Association, included 1,788 products sampled by hundreds of participants in ten locations. Generic Safeway, Wal-Mart, and other store brands far outranked name-brand counterparts. Generic raisin bran beat the national brands 62 to 28 percent. Bargain Hunters are immune to ads—except sale ads. They know that the mascara featured on that *Vogue* page will *not* make them prettier than cheap chain-store mascara.

Well, not *that* much prettier.

To Bargain Hunters, high prices simply seem *wrong*. Unethical. Unnecessary. Like some sort of trick. *What kind of moron*, Bargain Hunters ask, *would pay that much?* Bargain Hunters refuse to pay full price because they believe doing so is stupid. And again they might be right. After all, nearly half of American families spend more than they earn each year. The average American household carries some $8,000 in credit-card debt. And personal bankruptcies doubled between the 1990s and the 2000s. Wanting a secure future and knowing that every dollar counts, the Bargain Hunter is dead serious. Yet Bargain Hunters are among the world's most hated scavengers. This hatred is expressed subtly, via the raised eyebrow, the muttered comment, and the smirk. Consumer culture teaches that frugality is downright bad: that it is funny or sinister or even mean. *She's cheap; she doesn't want to share.* Compelled to join others at some restaurant or bar where they are expected to order from an expensive menu or share the group's tab, Bargain Hunters often feel intense discomfort. They feel cornered and defensive.

"I had to meet some former coworkers for dinner at a trendy

New Orleans–style restaurant," says our friend Ashley. "The place was packed. It was one of those places—like most places, I guess—where all the entrees are around fourteen bucks. To me that's a lot—I mean, just an entree; that doesn't include a salad or anything. At the buffet on the other side of town you get all you can eat for fourteen bucks. So I felt like an idiot paying that much for just a bowl of gumbo. Everyone else was totally cool with it. They were ordering like they do this all the time—well, they probably do—all excited, like they were actually looking forward to eating this expensive food, like they weren't thinking it was costing about fifty cents per bite. My turn came to order and I felt sick. Everyone was staring at me—they all knew, and I could see them trading these little glances like, 'There she goes again, the cheapskate.' And I couldn't do it. I couldn't order an entree. I just ordered a side dish of mashed potatoes. Of course the server said, 'Will that be all, Miss?' Their eyes were burning holes in me. I nodded yes.

"But the funny thing is—some of my ex-coworkers were facing financial difficulties. Two of them kept saying how hard-up and desperate they were for freelance work. And one said her husband had been laid off. Most of them are renters who don't like renting. They all wish they owned houses. I said, 'I just want to explain that when I order only a side dish here, it's not that I literally can't afford to order more—don't feel sorry for me, don't offer to pay for me. It's just that philosophically I don't believe in buying food that costs this much.' One woman blinked and said, 'Hmm, I never thought of this place as expensive.' And then they went on complaining about needing more work while ordering seven-dollar glasses of wine and eating their entrees in five minutes flat, then dessert. That was so weird to me."

Discount-Outlet Shopper

Quality-conscious yet open-minded and able to handle unpredictability, the Discount-Outlet Shopper greets every aisle with delight—like a butterfly touring a flower garden. *This* looks interesting! *That* looks tasty! *This* is organic! At these prices, buy six!

Discount grocery outlets sell food and other products—often in perfect condition, new, fresh, and sealed. They sell many of the exact same products from the exact same brands as are sold full price in ordinary stores—at about half the cost. This is because discount outlets acquire merchandise "opportunistically," as they say in the industry, snapping up "salvage"—that is, near-expiry closeouts, packaging misprints, liquidated goods from companies facing bankruptcy, labels that have been redesigned, and other overstock. Manufacturers would rather sell it supercheap by the palletload to discount outlets than throw it out or give it away for free. In other words, discount outlets are the scavengers of the grocery world.

A typical discount-outlet outfit, operating at least a hundred stores in six western states, is California-based Grocery Outlet, which calls itself the store "where you can actually save more money than you spend." Its founder began by buying military-surplus food and selling it under the name Cannery Sales, in 1946. Today, Grocery Outlet stores exude clean California-style cool, their wide aisles lined with the world's most recognizable brands—Coca-Cola, Kellogg's, and the like—along with local, ethnic, gourmet, and organic products. More and more such stores are giving standard-retail stores a run for their money.

Because discount outlets acquire stock opportunistically, their inventories are always in flux. Discount-Outlet Shoppers never know what they will find in the stores each time they visit. Yes, there will be juices. But will there be grape, pomegranate, *and* orange? Who knows? Discount-Outlet Shoppers are gamblers at heart: Buy a whole case of this imported Belgian chocolate now, or . . . just a box and hope some will be left when we come back? What if I buy three of these frozen vegan pizzas for a dollar-fifty each, eat one, and realize that it's the most delicious food I've ever tried? Should I buy five? What if I try one and despise it? Should I . . . ?

"Every trip to Grocery Outlet," reads a company promo, "is like a treasure hunt."

Coupon Clipper

Yo' mama's a scavenger. Right?

If she was one of those millions of homemakers who diligently clipped coupons from the grocery sections of daily newspapers, then yes. Underrecognized as a scavenger, the Coupon Clipper is a true American classic, combining the skills of a bargain hunter with those of a savvy planner. Coupon Clippers plan meals and menus in advance based on their coupon cull, then shop accordingly. Coupon Clippers are patient and thorough, now finding infinite new resources online, Googling "coupons" and "discounts" and "birthday deals." Champion Coupon Clippers organize their culls alphabetically, thematically, and/or by expiration date.

URBAN SCAVENGERS

The forms of scavenging detailed thus far all share one common feature. All involve payment. But other, wilder forms of scavenging involve *no money*. These aren't stealing. They aren't begging. But they all result in *getting stuff for free*.

Each form of free-stuff scavenging makes your mind work in brave new ways. A thrill infuses everything you see and do. A dare you set for yourself, for the world: *What can I get for free?*

Dumpster Diver

These days, Dumpster Divers are what come to mind when most people hear the word "scavenger." Dumpster Divers are the postmodern descendant of Édouard Manet's ragpicker, who wore dirty clothes and wielded a stick.

Some Dumpster Divers dive because they must, out of poverty. Yet a growing number dive by choice. Some are environmentalists. Many are anarchists. Scavenger-activists, they Dumpster-dive to get stuff but also to prove a point. They observe their own Dumpster Diver code of etiquette and they are, as a rule, polite. They dive by night, often in groups—for protection and to increase the yield, which is shared afterward. And some dive by day.

Long epitomized as bottom-feeders, Dumpster Divers are becoming thoroughly assimilated into the mainstream as people of all kinds now feel comfortable admitting that they dive. "I love to Dumpster-dive. People throw away perfectly good stuff that others can use," writes a boomer at Boomertowne.com. "I love to Dumpster dive and I mean peek inside the big green monster, poke around with a stick and grab what appeals to me," writes Dawn at QueerCents.com. "I love to Dumpster dive! . . . I got about 400 dollars worth of lotion, perfume, powder and makeup. I wear my oldest clothes when I go," explains a Kentucky mom at Frugalvillage.com. California interior designer and TV talk-show host Carol Tanzi, who calls herself "the Goddess of Garbage" and creates artworks with Dumpster finds, uses as her logo a cartoon of herself emerging from a bright yellow Dumpster wielding a flower bouquet. "Find a dumpster," urges the community wiki for Davis, California. "Climb in, and search for something useful. Some amazing things can be found in dumpsters in this town." The wiki lists "trash temples"—that is, prime Dumpsters in which to find books, furniture, and food. (The latter category includes bakeries, supermarkets, candy shops, and cinemas.) Dumpster diving is a popular theme at the social-networking site Meetup .com, with groups such as the five-hundred-member New York City Dumpster Diving Meetup Group, whose calendar of events includes "Trash Trailblaze in Ridgeway, Queens." Members of the Nashville group call themselves "Dumpstranauts." In Seattle, they're "Dumpster Divas," and they invite interested females to "meet other fun, fabulous (and otherwise normal) ladies interested in sustainable living, salvaging, reusing, repurposing and having fun. This group is open to all non-radical, socially conscious women concerned about wastefulness and reducing their impact, regardless of dumpster experience. Beginners and experienced divers encouraged to join."

Dumpster Divers are bolder than most, have higher "ick" thresholds, and are not claustrophobic. Yes, you can Dumpster "dive" by standing on the ground outside a Dumpster and poking through its contents with a stick. (A stick with a hook attached to one end is especially handy.) But the true Dumpster Diver climbs inside. This means becoming, at least for a time, part of its contents.

You become one with the trash.

And you're cocooned. Confined. Enclosed. Encased. You cannot get out easily. When you are Dumpster diving, you cannot pretend to be doing something else.

Dumpsters are trash receptacles. Thus they can be gross, slimy, even dangerous inside. You might find spoiled food, biohazards, broken glass. You might find the contents of the used-tampon bins from the employee restroom. Dumpster Divers sometimes wear gloves. Many bring bandages and antiseptic.

Dumpster diving for forty years, our friend Ralph still dives at age seventy-six. Anyone seeing this wiry white-haired figure parking his bike beside a Dumpster and hoisting himself over the side will assume, Ralph laughs, "that I'm a homeless bum." Nothing could be further from the truth. He has a comfortable home and recently retired. Ralph's favorite Dumpster is behind a grocery store. The amount of food he finds there never ceases to astound him. (And rightly so. According to the California Integrated Waste Management Board, more than 150,000 tons of food are thrown away every year in Alameda County, where Ralph lives.) Ralph buys rice and beans regularly. He scavenges everything else he eats.

"Before you go into any store," he advises, "just step over to its Dumpster and look inside. Maybe you'll find in there what you were about to go inside and buy. Maybe you'll find a loaf of bread—okay, a day old, but so what? Maybe you'll find some only slightly blemished apples. We're a throwaway society."

FREE-Box Forager

Because his sole mode of transportation is a bicycle, Ralph spends much of his time outdoors on residential streets, where he finds many objects set out on curbs and sidewalks bearing FREE signs. Also on curbs and sidewalks, he finds FREE boxes—whole cartons full of discarded items, placed there by their former owners and marked FREE.

FREE boxes are a localized tradition. Some areas have none,

while in others, such as the San Francisco area where Ralph lives, they're a ubiquitous hippie-era legacy. Some towns even have *permanent* FREE boxes, large wooden constructions where locals drop off unwanted items for others to collect. Because of its shape and sheltering roof, one such box in Berkeley is called the Wishing Well. A municipal FREE box has been a landmark in the California beach town of Bolinas since 1974. Most FREE boxes, however, are spontaneous and temporary: someone's moving out of an apartment, someone's decluttering a bookcase or kitchen or closet. Into a cardboard box the items go, onto the curb. Finders keepers.

Free-Box Foragers love surprises. They expect nothing, so every free box they encounter is a plus, even if it is empty by the time they reach it. For the Free-Box Forager, it's almost enough just to know *free stuff was here. Someone else got it, but this box is proof that there is free stuff out there in the world and sometimes it's for me.*

Every FREE box is like a surprise grab bag, the ultimate example of that scavenging adage: *You never know.* Not only can you never know whether you will encounter any FREE boxes on any given outing, you also cannot know where they might be or what might be inside them. More than nearly every other scavenging venue, FREE boxes are a matter of sheer luck.

This is what makes them so exciting. You do not (because you cannot) seek them. You find them unbidden, in your path. No matter what turns out to be inside, just the thrill of spotting a box, spying that word FREE from down the block, around the corner, or across the street, feels like your birthday, feels like Chanukah or Christmas, feels like you've stumbled over treasure, feels like someone smiled and said, "Here—catch!" Draw closer and your blood races. You do not know yet whether it contains a single bent paper clip or a fully functional fax machine or a still-sealed bottle of South African marula-fruit liqueur. You do not know yet whether it contains a drill set or a teapot or the 1986 back issues of *Soldier of Fortune* magazine. You do not know yet whether it contains Legos or lithographs of what looks like the Alps. You do not know yet whether it contains a blender or a silver bracelet or the one thing in the world that will now and forever be what you love most of all. You do not know.

But that's the point.

You do not know.

Free Marketer

Free markets are part flea market and part yard sale and part swap, imbued with the gleeful communitarian anarchism of the freegan movement (see page 176). Because the free market is a comparatively new venue, free markets occur only in a few selected cities—as yet.

The Craigslist.org ad for one in San Francisco reads: "Really Really Free Market. Bring whatever you don't want anymore. And TAKE whatever you DO want. For FREE!!!" The organizers host free markets in the city's Dolores Park once a month. One Saturday, they spread sheets over the grass as hipsters arrive in ones and twos. Some of them empty backpacks and shopping bags onto the sheets, unloading clothes and other stuff to give away. Others stroll from sheet to sheet, snatching items and slinging them over their shoulders or into backpacks of their own. Lacy dress. Yoink! Sealed box of different-sized screwdrivers: Thank you very much. Vintage vinyl Jefferson Airplane album: Nab. Black leather jacket, sleeves scuffed only a bit. A perfect fit, I'll wear it home. For Free Marketers, it's a two-handed process: unpack your own discards with one hand while snatching someone else's with the other. Some make a day of it, circling slowly, waiting for new arrivals, time and again venturing back. The air is one of generosity and opportunity. You keep forgetting that these people grinning and pressing their old swimsuits into your hand as you give them your child's outgrown car seat are not friends but total strangers, united in scavenging. You feel almost naughty, like you're trading secret wisdom, too.

Finder

Finders do not seek. Not consciously. Not pointedly. Finders *find.*

They have a gift. Most Finders discovered this gift as little kids. They were the ones who saw what no one else noticed: the nickel in the sand, the ripe blackberries growing up a wall. Others teased them: *Do you have eyes in the back of your head?*

Yes, and in their arms, their derrieres, their feet. Finders find diamonds in snowdrifts, iPods in the tall grass under park benches, five-dollar bills slotted in books. All other types of scavenging are forms of finding. But Finders are primal, somewhat spiritual scavengers, because what they find, while usually welcome, is *always* unsought and unexpected. For the Finder, finding is a way of getting stuff but also an ongoing game. A test. A form of divination: What will the cosmos give me today? Ah: I found this. Here. Now. *Why* this? *Why* here? *Why* now? *Why* me? What might it mean?

Asked where he or she got that necklace, flute, or oil painting, the Finder shrugs: *I found it.*

At first, nobody believes.

Aftermather

When the county fair is over, when the crowds have left, when the yard sale is over, and when the flea market is over . . . stuff almost always remains. It fell to the ground unnoticed. Or it was left outside, marked FREE. Or it was chucked into the nearest trash bin.

Aftermathers gather this detritus. Sifting through what is lost and unwanted and abandoned from the sites where others haggled over what was already lost and unwanted and abandoned, After-mathers scavenge after scavengers. Some see themselves as saviors, reminding their finds: Between you and total abandonment, there is *only me.*

Urban Gleaner

Fresh, delicious free food isn't as hard to find as you might think. Sometimes it literally grows on trees.

The Urban Gleaner is an amateur horticulturalist, able to identify fruit-bearing trees and bushes by their leaves and branches, even out of season. Urban Gleaners know where to go to pick what when.

Urban Gleaners study up on which types of fruit ripen during which weeks or months in their areas. Depending on what they learn from personal experience and websites, Urban Gleaners locate examples of those trees and bushes growing in (or extending over) public areas such as sidewalks and parking lots. The community wiki for Davis, California, helpfully maps out apple trees along a bike path, pomegranate trees in an apartment-house parking lot, and loquat and apricot trees between university lecture halls. Urban Gleaners observe a certain etiquette: Don't break branches and don't pick on private property without permission. Always carry spare plastic bags during fruit seasons. When you find an especially bountiful tree, fill the bags; when you get home, prepare and freeze the fruit. (Peaches and plums, for example, freeze best when halved and pitted.) Some parts of the country are so fertile, with so many produce-bearing trees and bushes planted so long ago as to now be fully mature, that Urban Gleaners in those areas need never actually pay for a single fruit again.

Founded by a group of artists in Los Angeles and dedicated to "the liberation of public fruit," the Fallen Fruit collective advocates urban gleaning. Its events include the Public Fruit Jam—a free annual jam-making session in Echo Park—and moonlight picking strolls through fruit-tree-rich neighborhoods, the Silver Lake district in summer for loquats, for instance. According to its manifesto, Fallen Fruit's goal is to make use of "all the free fruit we can find. Every day there is food somewhere going to waste. We encourage you to find it, tend and harvest it. If you own property, plant food on your perimeter. Share with the world and the world will share with you. Barter, don't buy! Give things away! You have nothing to lose but your hunger!"

While sunny Los Angeles is blessed with plentiful fruit trees, the collective laments the sparse urban-gleaning resources elsewhere.

"A specter is haunting our cities," mourns the manifesto. "Barren landscapes with foliage and flowers, but nothing to eat. Fruit can grow almost anywhere, and can be harvested by everyone. Our cities are planted with frivolous and ugly landscaping, sad shrubs and neglected trees, whereas they should burst with ripe produce. Great sums of money are spent on young trees, water and maintenance. While these trees are beautiful, they could be healthy, fruitful and beautiful. We ask all of you to petition your cities and towns to support community gardens and only plant fruit-bearing trees in public parks. Let our streets be lined with apples and pears! Demand that all parking lots be landscaped with fruit trees which provide shade, clean the air and feed the people."

(Urban Gleaners are only distantly related to Rural Gleaners, discussed later in this chapter.)

Library Lizard

Library Lizards scavenge very quietly. And they look smart. They are another classic, unsung type of scavenger. We've all heard anecdotes about famous people who spent much of their youth in public libraries, where (often with the help of kindly librarians) they discovered the book or the subject that eventually shaped their illustrious careers. Any section of any library is a scavenger's paradise. Library Lizards scavenge entertainment, pastimes, and the most valuable treasure of all: information.

Heck, why even buy books? Granted, that is not a question we should be asking in a book, but libraries make paying to read anything, *ever*, seem patently ridiculous. Library Lizards read for free. Library Lizards check out DVDs and videos to watch at home for free. They use materials borrowed from libraries to learn, create, achieve.

On cold and rainy days, homeless Library Lizards scavenge shelter there.

Recycling Poacher

Ever since municipal recycling programs began, a certain predatory type of scavenger has been giving the rest of us a bad rap. Usually in the predawn hours, usually pulling noisy shopping carts, Recycling Poachers ramble from house to house, sometimes staying on the curb but sometimes walking up private driveways and even into yards. Collecting glass, plastic, and paper from household recycling bins, they later sell it at recycling centers.

Laws regarding this practice vary from place to place. Sometimes the poaching of recyclables counts as a public nuisance, sometimes as theft. On private property, it's trespassing. Recycling companies are authorized to collect recyclables in their trucks in counties, cities, and neighborhoods. Recycling Poachers are stealing from those authorized recyclers. Yes, Recycling Poachers are often poor and must survive on whatever they get for what they find. But legally dubious scavenging makes outsiders believe the worst of all of us, so that when they hear the word "scavenger," they think of shabby figures scuttling up their driveways and through their gates in the dark.

In some areas, under certain circumstances, Recycling Poachers can be arrested and fined.

SOCIAL SCAVENGERS

Freecycler (and Internet-Free-Stuff Trader)

Freecyclers are pen pals who *give each other free stuff.*

The word "freecycle" is often used conversationally to mean a process by which people post online items they wish to give away, and others request and receive those items, free. One might say: "I freecycled this guitar."

But the word derives from Freecycle.org, the world's biggest scavenging network. You might not know the mom-of-three who lives twelve blocks away from you on the north side of town and works at the bike-repair shop, but she's giving away a color printer and you want it and you'll get it. You might not know the college student who just moved into one of those apartments over the pizzeria across the street from campus, but he's about to get that yellow couch you don't want anymore. You do not know each other, yet you are fellow Freecyclers.

Organized into thousands of regional chapters in more than seventy-five countries, Freecycle.org was founded in 2003 on the premise that landfills could be reduced if people gave stuff away rather than threw it out. Now it has chapters in Cameroon, Oman, the Cayman Islands, and just about every other place you can think of; its motto is "Changing the world one gift at a time."

Other gifting groups have arisen as well. Some are one-offs but others are chains such as FreeBay (like eBay, but free), CurbCycle, ReUseIt, Recycle4Free, Around Again, and Sharing Is Giving. More than nine hundred such groups throughout the English-speaking world are registered at the Freesharing.org portal—from Calgary Treasure Hunters to Wise County, Texas rEcycle ("Rich or poor makes no difference at all, for all are welcome here") to Janesville Gently Loved to SydneyTrashNTreasure to RealCycle Bedfordshire to Give and Take West Midlands. Anderson (South Carolina) Foodshare is devoted solely to the exchange of "perishable or nonperishable unexpired/unspoiled food items that might otherwise go to waste," including "excess items from government programs ... from your cabinets and pantries, seeds, plants, fruit before it rots on the tree, excess veggies from the farm or garden, canned goods ... pet foods, and so on." The level of commitment is palpable. "If anyone tries to charge you in any way, please report it," warn the Coos Bay (Oregon) Free Circle People. Glasgow Freeshare, just one group in one city, boasts more than 10,000 members. Freecycling also thrives at general classified-ad sites such as Craigslist.org.

The size and number of these groups are dazzling proof of a major social shift now afoot. History has turned a corner. Rendering full-price retail all the more marginal, freecycling makes scavenging easier than ever. We can scavenge in the comfort of our own homes with just a click.

Freecyclers are sociable, and these groups are a new type of social unit: welcoming, supportive, loyal, tribal, and proud.

"WANTED: table fountain, toaster oven, whistling teapot, etc.," a member of the Berkeley Freecycle group writes briskly. "Just moved into an apartment"—the neighborhood he cites is rather affluent—"and am looking for a few things: Valances (2, those things that decorate the tops of windows). Tabletop wine rack for 5–8 bottles. Tapestry to cover a nasty door. . . . Coffee Maker. Teapot (that whistles).

"If any of you have any of these," this Freecycler writes, "that'd be wonderful."

Freegan

Embracing a name that merges "free" with "vegan," Freegans belong to a proud new sociopolitical movement, forging a lifestyle that manifests their beliefs and principles. Radical anticonsumerists, Freegans boycott all aspects of the standard profit-driven economy, which they believe is unethical and harmful to people, animals, and the Earth. In other words, they aim to live without spending a cent. As such, they rank among the most dedicated full-time scavengers of all. Avid Dumpster divers, Freegans devise ingenious alternative means of finding, foraging, and trading. One well-known Freegan-inspired group is Food Not Bombs. Founded in Massachusetts in the 1980s and now boasting some four hundred chapters in at least sixty countries, FNB is a network of anarchist-activist collectives that demonstrate their antiestablishmentarianism by cooking and serving free vegan or vegetarian meals weekly to all takers in public sites such as parks.

Most of the ingredients come from surplus donated by companies and stores; some come from Dumpsters. Each chapter is independent, with its own website listing serving times and places. Although, overall, FNB is antiwar and anticonsumerist, each chapter has its own special slant. FNB's Guatemala chapter promises to "feed immediately those people who lack adequate food," and to "reinstate a system whose priorities are to empower and satisfy the necessities of all human beings."

The Freegan philosophy also advocates squatting (because Freegans believe housing is a right, not a privilege), hitchhiking, healing illnesses with wild plants, and working as little as possible (because virtually all companies are part of the system). While ordinary urban freeganism is already pretty extreme by most standards, some Freegans "go feral"—setting up survivalist scavenger outposts in the wilderness.

Clothing Swapper

Are you the type who always used to borrow your siblings' clothes? The type who, when complimenting someone's outfit, really, truly *wants* that outfit? You're a Clothing Swapper.

The swapping movement began in the '90s as a reaction to high retail prices and as a creative way to shed all those why-did-I-buy-this mistakes and all those wrong-color-wrong-style-wrong-size gifts received from clueless loved ones—and get stuff in exchange.

Organized with friends, neighbors, coworkers, or total strangers, a swap is a party to which every guest brings at least one item—sometimes many more—to give away. The manner of redistribution is up to you. Some make it into fun games: drawing lots, mock auctions, Easter-egg-type hunts, musical chairs as guests seize the nearest items when the music stops, Let's Make a Deal as guests are asked to perform bizarre ordeals to win wrapped mystery items, Twenty Questions as each guest holds his or her item hidden inside a bag or box. Other swappers simply sit in a circle and pass their items to whomever is seated to their right or left. Others make a debate of it, with all items displayed and each guest making an impassioned plea for the item he or she most desires; when two or more guests compete for the same item, the other guests pick a winner by secret ballot. Some swaps are impromptu flea markets, with guests "selling" each other their items. And some swaps, of course, are free-for-alls.

Free-Sample Forager (and Reception Habitué)

Free-Sample Foragers and Reception Habitués scavenge their way to lavish repasts. Hot food samples are sometimes served at your favorite supermarket. Free lectures are often accompanied by free receptions, open to the public. Receptions also often accompany art gallery openings.

Free-Sample Foragers and Reception Habitués search classifieds and local calendars for events that might have free food. In college towns, the adept Reception Habitué could easily go a whole week at a stretch without either cooking or buying a meal.

But detective work is only the beginning. Much sample foraging and *all* reception cruising include a social element. At stores, one chats with sample servers. At receptions, one mingles with fellow attendees. Receptions are basically parties, but unnatural in the sense that attendees tend to be total strangers to each other. Some Reception Habitués eat and run, or fill their paper plates with free food and run, eating it later. (Not that we recommend this.) Staying at the reception means almost certainly being compelled to talk to strangers. About what? The art being exhibited, or the lecture accompanying the reception, is the best bet. A loner? Become absorbed in the art, in the view out the window or the books lining the shelves.

There is, admittedly, an embarrassment factor. Not everyone feels comfortable taking advantage of all the free food the social scene has to offer. Free-Sample Foragers sometimes feel like thieves and Reception Habitués feel like party crashers. But no. *Businesses give away free food all the time.* It's part of successful marketing campaigns. And ethical Reception Habitués attend only events that *are* free and open to the public. (Sneaking into private fetes or paid events *is* similar to theft, however, so we don't encourage it.)

Free-Sample Foragers and Reception Habitués are pragmatists. Whatever comes their way, they eat. *Beggars,* they quip, though they never beg, *can't be choosers.*

No-Cost Gardener (and Seed Swapper)

Gardening can be an expensive pastime. Calculate the standard retail cost of plants and seeds and soil and chemicals and tools. It's enough to make you think of paving over your yard.

Yet even a single flower, vegetable, or fruit can produce a whole handful of seeds—enough to grow a whole bed. And every garden has dozens of flowers, vegetables, and/or fruits. You eat and walk past hundreds more each day. Why pay for seeds?

No-Cost Gardeners scavenge seeds wherever they go. Local ecology centers in some cities have "seed exchange" areas, where No-Cost Gardeners can collect seeds (and bulbs and rhizomes) of their choosing from labeled jars or drawers, and/or donate seeds of their own. The Bay Area Seed Interchange Library

(BASIL), as a good example, invites gardeners to freely take (or donate) as many seeds as they like from a kaleidoscopic array that eclipses the selection in most retail outlets. Seed Swappers also meet and trade online—and at a kind of confab that has become increasingly common since 1989, when gardening groups in Canada and Great Britain started staging official "Seedy Saturday" and "Seedy Sunday" swaps in order to increase biodiversity and sustain heritage varieties. The United States followed suit with "National Seed Swap Day," celebrated on the last Saturday in January. But community seed swaps—which are essentially horticultural free markets—happen year-round. An invitation to a typical swap in Oakland, California, exhorts: "Instant new garden! Bring your plants and pick up new ones. Have plants you must prune or cull?" it asks. "How about trading your excess with others in your neighborhood? All types and sizes of plants welcome—small cuttings up to full size specimens, seeds & bulbs, herbs and vegetables. Gardening accessories, tools and supplies welcome, too." A list of the latter includes "stepping stones, trellises, pots, stakes, driftwood, compost bins, weed whackers, goldfish, lawnmowers, and yard art."

We, the authors, have maintained a no-cost garden for years, scavenging not only exotic and rare seeds for intriguing harvests but all the other supplies—trowels, buckets, and so on—used for urban farming.

SPECIALTY SCAVENGERS

A far cry from those who scavenge to survive, specialty scavengers are hobbyists following their hopes and dreams, spanning a wide range of interests and goals.

Metal Detector

It looks like nothing more than a disk or a ring attached to one end of a long rod, but a metal detector has the seemingly magical capacity to detect the presence of metals on or under the ground at various distances depending on its strength. The user—who, awkwardly, is also called a metal detector—arcs it back and forth ahead of him as he walks over flat ground or sand.

And therein lie ten million fantasies.

Police use metal detectors to investigate crime scenes. And some hobbyists and scholars seek valuable artifacts and antiques. We'll discuss these in a moment. But many scavengers use metal detectors to seek contemporary coins, jewelry, and other fairly new objects. An hour spent detecting at a beach, school yard, or park—the three most popular detecting sites—might typically yield a pocketful of pull tabs, nails, several coins new and old, and an earring or two. But it's the process that counts, and the promise: in this processed world, metal detecting is our version of unearthing buried treasure. Two shiny dimes and a bottle cap and a bent Izod zipper pull found one to seven inches under the soil of a school playground? It's the thought that counts.

Well, not really. It's finding stuff that counts, and the best kind of stuff is not only valuable, but old and mysterious, reeking of secrets and forgotten stories. On a recent metal-detecting foray to an empty lot, we dug up in one afternoon: a broken silver-and-amber bracelet, an antique key, a lead fishing weight stamped with Chinese characters, a collar tag for a dog named "Sumi," a quarter stained a bizarre shade of purple, a rusted drill bit, some aluminum foil, a 1932 circular tin box for holding Three Cadet brand condoms (far and away the best find of the day), $1.37 in change, an ugly button, a 1966 ten-pence coin from Jamaica, a solid silver casino token "redeemable for seven dollars" at the Reno Circus

Circus, and more nails, bolts, bottle caps, and soda cans than we care to mention.

Sound fun? Then metal detecting is for you.

Before getting started, check with local treasure-hunting clubs about regulations regarding metal detecting in your area. Digging up grass is usually illegal in public parks, for instance. And never treasure-hunt on private property without permission. You might want to join that treasure-hunting club. Most offer group activities such as day trips and contests, and publish newsletters announcing new machine technologies and interesting finds. Then again, if you're the jealous type who would seethe if your companion found a diamond ring two feet away from you, then *do not join.* Metal detecting is arguably best enjoyed alone.

Beaches are optimal sources for finding rings because fingers, already lubricated by sunscreen and suntan oil, shrink when immersed in cold water. Beaches in areas that are favorite honeymoon destinations are best, because brand-new rings tend not to fit well.

Even finding items that are far from antique evokes a sense of wonder. Describing his latest finds in a film posted at YouTube.com, a hobbyist named Steve declares, "Everything that's found is a moment in time. . . . I found two lovely gold rings and I thought to myself: . . . All those little winter nights sitting there on their own . . . and now they're back in the sunshine and that's just great. . . . It's nice when you hold it in your hand and you feel: *Well, that could've been lost forever.* You feel like you're sort of the guardian of it again."

Beachcomber

Beaches are where wild nature and fun-seeking humanity often meet. The result is a glorious, ever-changing array of scavengeable treasures both natural and human-made, delivered in the most dramatic setting possible. Finding nice things along a shore—whether it's driftwood or seashells or coins—feels magical, like having been tossed a prize from an undersea kingdom. The authors of this book once spent a winter living a few blocks from a Pacific Ocean beach. Although summer is obviously the best time to beachcomb for just-lost coins and jewelry, winter is best for strange, storm-tossed marvels cast ashore by the waves.

Over that winter, we found surf-smoothed moonstones and agates, enough to fill ten jars. We found festoons of plastic fishing floats from Korea. A life preserver bearing stenciled Russian words. Wooden-handled savage hooks used to drag tuna and other large fish on deck. But what we found most of, and what was *not* included in our childhood beachcombing fantasy, was trash. Actual garbage—toothpaste tubes, plastic scrubbers, dish-soap bottles, shampoo bottles, soft-drink bottles, toilet brushes, cans. But it was interesting trash, washed clean by the wide ocean, with labels that bore the languages of the world: Tagalog, Polish, Hindi, German, Japanese, Arabic, Chinese, English, Thai, Russian, Portuguese—the discards of a thousand fishing boats and cargo ships, chucked overboard. Millions of tons of solid waste float on the sea. A bit of it washed up that year in Oregon. Some of the bottles seemed quite old, having circled the Pacific for decades before finding their way to our beach. Fascinated, we gathered the international trash in bags and brought it home. We still keep some of it as souvenirs.

Modern-day Beachcombers bear witness to human wastefulness in all its horror. This has led to the birth of a new form of scavenging: the beach cleanup. Municipalities and nonprofits host these cleanups regularly, urging the public to volunteer and offering free coffee and snacks to all participants. Often a representative from an environmentalist group gives a talk on oceanic

ecology and explains the dire effects of ocean-borne trash. On
Beach Cleanup Day 2008—September 20—some 55,000 volunteers collected about 742,000 pounds of trash from California
beaches. *That much, in just one day.*

Treasure Hunter

The idea of going out and discovering riches—not working for
them or even winning them but *finding* them—has been an ultimate human fantasy ever since the first hominid bent down to
pick up a pretty rock. Unlike other forms of scavenging that celebrate minimalism and thrift, treasure hunting is all about un-
imaginable wealth awaiting the lucky and the plucky. Sending
chills down the spine, treasure-hunting tales are cracking yarns,
swashbuckling sagas about lost mines, ghost towns, sunken ships,
buried chests, ingots, El Dorado, pirate caverns ashine with emeralds and pearls. In many such tales, scavenging turns into larceny or plunder. In many, treasure is a metaphor for greed and
incivility: finders betray each other, refuse to reveal a cache, and
die rather than share. In Alexandre Dumas's *The Count of Monte
Cristo*, a dying priest confides to his fellow prisoner, a young sailor,
the secret location of a huge hidden treasure "in the caves of the
small island of Monte Cristo . . . ingots, gold, money, jewels, diamonds, gems . . . which may amount to two millions of Roman
crowns, and which he will find on raising the twentieth rock from
the small creek to the east." After escaping prison in the old man's
body bag, the sailor makes his way to the islet. Finding the treasure, "he then closed his eyes as children do in order to perceive
in the shining night of their own imagination more stars than are
visible in the firmament." There at his feet "blazed piles of golden
coin. . . . Edmond grasped handfuls of diamonds, pearls, and ru-
bies, which as they fell on one another sounded like hail against

glass. . . . Edmond rushed through the caverns like a man seized with frenzy." Aided by his incalculable new riches, the sailor returns incognito to France, where posing as an aristocrat he wreaks revenge on his enemies. The revenge goes too far and fills him with regret.

But sometimes the treasure isn't metaphorical at all. Sometimes it's real.

We've all seen the headlines: "Treasure-Laden Shipwreck Found off African Coast." "Deep-Sea Booty! 500 Million in Coins Found." "4,100-Year-Old Treasure Found in Bulgaria." "15th Century Shipwreck Laden with Treasure Found." (And yes, those headlines are real, appearing on NationalGeographic.com, MSNBC.com, and CNN.com.) Impossible as it sounds, astounding hoards are still being discovered by archaeologists, professional salvaging teams, and amateurs alike. This is scavenging on a grand scale, and a single search often consumes years of effort and millions of dollars. The lucky European amateur Treasure Hunter using a metal detector in a historical area sometimes happens upon buried Viking or Saxon hoards—and, depending on the treasure-trove laws in the country where the find is made, sometimes gets to keep it.

Prospector

The great gold rushes of the nineteenth century created a stereotypical image of the Prospector: a wizened, straggly-whiskered stick of a creature with a look of crazed determination, wielding a pickax. Rich and colorful legendry surrounds this rough-hewn, risk-embracing, all-American version of the Treasure Hunter. Yet Prospectors are not wholly a thing of the past. The lure of striking it rich by hewing minerals or precious metals from the Earth still sends many professionals and amateurs into the creeks, rivers, and hills. Nationwide financial crises further reinforce this lure. If the banks fail, says the Prospector, I'll have gold. With higher-tech equipment such as automatic gold-panning machines being developed, Prospectors constitute a vibrant community, which even has its own jokes:

Q: Why did the prospector throw his ore samples away?
A: He took them for granite.
Q: Why did the prospector make his mom carry his ore samples?
A: He thought it was the mother lode.

The stereotypical pickax-wielding icon appears on the websites of many modern prospecting clubs. One such club, the Gold Prospectors Association of America, sponsors digs, reviews prospecting equipment, and sells instructional DVDs. An invitation to a group dig begins with a close-up of a right hand emptying a vial of nuggets into a left palm, as huge words spread across the screen: WOULD. YOU. LIKE. TO. FIND. GOLD??? A voice chimes in: "Well, here's your chance!" The camera pans over a hillside where dozens of hobbyists are wielding metal detectors and picks. "Potluck! Bonfires! Fun for the whole family! . . . We'll see ya there, pardner."

Professional Archaeologist

At least one branch of academia lets its members make careers out of scavenging. With the generous backing of their universities, along with the sponsorship of historical societies, national governments, and other institutions, Professional Archaeologists get to travel the world digging and diving for stuff. Through their efforts, museums fill up with marvels, teaching us almost everything we know about the rise and fall of cities and civilizations. Perhaps the findings of these scholar-scavengers will someday teach us enough to keep our civilization from falling, too.

Amateur Archaeologist

All scavenging is archaeology, really. Even a found McDonald's cup dropped ten minutes ago is archaeology. Amateur Archaeologists want more. With no sponsorship, no credentials, and no teams of interns eager to do the dirty work, Amateur Archaeologists love history. They also love the zest of a treasure hunt. Researching local history with the help of books, the Internet, historical societies, and hearsay, they mount their own expeditions in whatever promising places-with-a-past that they can find: the field behind the old church, say, or the waste ground that used to be a drive-in theater. Construction or road-repair sites in historic areas have been known to yield artifacts that literally slipped between the cracks of former buildings or slipped beneath the dusty surfaces of former (unpaved) roads.

The conscientious Amateur Archaeologist bones up beforehand on local laws regarding access and digging, and *never* metal-detects on private property without permission. Upon learning that a certain private property such as farmland or the backyard of a house has a historically rich past, the Amateur Archaeologist can make arrangements with its owner, offering the owner a percentage of whatever might be found in exchange for permission to search there.

Rural Gleaner

In her 2000 documentary *The Gleaners and I*, French filmmaker Agnès Varda tags along with various types of scavengers, urban and rural, to record their tactics and philosophy. The film's title derives from Varda's first and most compelling subjects, Rural Gleaners, who go in groups to collect whatever has been left behind in potato fields, apple orchards, and vineyards after the official harvest has been brought in. As discussed earlier in this book, this practice is detailed in the Old Testament, which tells farmers: "When you reap the harvest of your land, you shall not reap your field to its very border, neither shall you gather the gleanings after your harvest. And you shall not strip your vineyard bare, neither shall you gather the fallen grapes of your vineyard; you shall leave them for the poor" (Leviticus 19:9–10 RSV). The film's title also alludes to Jean-François Millet's famous 1857 painting depicting three women gathering sheaves and kernels in a golden wheat field under a pink-blue sky. Collecting produce that has been left behind because it is the wrong size or shape, the film's Rural Gleaners are individualistic, pragmatic, realistic. Plucking an apple that clearly isn't pretty enough for retail, one quips: "This apple is like a stupid ugly woman: zero value." Some are desperately poor; others glean on principle.

Most Rural Gleaners today belong to humanitarian groups like the Virginia-based Society of St. Andrew, whose volunteers arrange to gather millions of pounds of postharvest grain and produce from American agricultural outfits every year, then distribute it to the needy. But in some specialized agricultural regions, such as the wine-growing Sonoma and Napa valleys of California, independent individuals love to glean the leftover fruit after the harvest to make jam, chutney, and even liqueur.

Found-Object Artist

Technically, the first Found-Object Artists were prehistoric cave dwellers creating ritual objects and wall paintings with scavenged sticks, stones, skins, feathers, ocher, and mud. Although such works went out of style in the civilized West for many millennia, they reemerged with Marcel Duchamp, the French Dadaist who (as already mentioned) early in the twentieth century exhibited such quotidian objects as a bicycle wheel and a urinal, choosing the name "readymades" for this then startling series. Another term for this kind of work, *assemblage*, was coined in the 1950s by the French artist Jean Dubuffet, who used scrap wood, scrap paper, sponges, and other found materials to create three-dimensional collages. From the highest echelons of the art and design worlds to the kindergarten classroom, Found-Object Artists have proliferated ever since, their inspirations ranging from back-to-the-land pastoralism to environmentalism to nihilism.

In 2005, Berlin's Gallery twenty-four per website hosted the International Assemblage Artist Exhibition. Among the works by sixty-five artists from thirty-seven different countries were a wall-mounted ironing board with light fixtures attached; a collage with bottle caps affixed over the breasts of a woman in a vintage photograph; and a painted seascape with sardine cans and scrap fishnet attached. The rapidly expanding craftster movement is home to countless Found-Object Artists. More than any other type of scavenger, Found-Object Artists give scavenging a cool, hip image that smashes old stereotypes and silences would-be critics. Salvaging consumer waste, a growing number of design companies merge found-object art with green-movement commitment. Brooklyn-based RePlayGround makes clocks out of computer keyboards, coffee tables out of car windows, and sells ReMakeIt kits: just add your own scrap.

San Francisco's sanitation facility, SF Recycling and Disposal, operates an Artist in Residence program in which local artists are allotted a monthly stipend and twenty-four-hour access to a 2,000-square-foot studio at the dump, where they create art using materials they have salvaged from the forty-four-acre site. At the end of each artist's residency, the artworks are displayed at exhibitions that draw enthusiastic crowds. Artworks made during the course of the program are then exhibited in office buildings and public spaces throughout the city.

In September 2008, the dump's Artist in Residence was Casey Logan, whose works employed such elements as scrap wood, audio speakers, globes, and toy planes.

IN ÉDOUARD MANET'S DAY, the artist painted the ragpicker. The artist *is* the ragpicker today.

CHAPTER 7

LAND OF
THE FREE

Living Thriftily

WHY BOTHER?

Scavenging is work. It saves us money, but it's work.

And shopping for brand-new stuff, at full price, is *eeeeeasy.* Not only do advertisements permeate our lives, telling us exactly what to buy and where and how and hinting that, without it, we will be hideous and alone, consumer culture has created new, improved technologies for buying all that stuff. *Right. Now.* ATMs rear up everywhere. Kids as young as ten use debit cards designed especially for them with cool names like Buxx and UPside. When money from parents' accounts is deposited automatically into their children's "allowance accounts," the children can withdraw it whenever they like, without having to tell the folks what for.

Click.

"As your parents will tell you," reads a Buxx Card promo,

"it's never too early to start spending responsibly and saving for your future."

Riiiight.

"Find out how to find the best ways to pay for purchases and stay financially healthy."

Mm-hmmm.

The best way to save for your future and stay financially healthy is to *not* spend money. But consumer culture won't tell you that, because consumer culture has stuff to sell you. Right. Now.

With so much stuff out there, and so many ways of acquiring it instantly, scavenging is a workout. It requires skills, will, patience, perseverance. Full-time scavenging, even part-time scavenging, means thinking and acting in whole new ways. It means excising truisms that have been seared into your brain. It means relinquishing, maybe forever, luxuries you took for granted. This will feel awful at first. It will feel like withdrawal. One day you will tell yourself: *I'm here freezing without a coat and Macy's is across the street and I will not go in. Am I an idiot?* Being a scavenger means turning your values inside out. It means stopping to think at moments when you never would have thought before. Being a scavenger means going out into the world and doing things that others might scorn. Then *doing them again*, and being proud.

That's hard. So—why go to all that effort?

You know. You have your reasons. So do all scavengers.

To save money.

To save the Earth.

To protest wastefulness.

To protest high prices because a twenty-seven-dollar dish of ravioli in a restaurant seems literally criminal to you.

To protest conformity because you cannot stand the thought

of looking like everyone else and looking like some corporate hack decided you should look.

To avoid becoming a spoiled indebted narcissist.

Fill in your other reasons here.

So now you're thinking: *I'm convinced. I have my reasons and I want to make the change. But how?*

Well, troop—

This is scavenging boot camp.

Yes, it is entirely possible to get for free or nearly free almost anything you want or require.

It is entirely possible to live for days on end without spending a cent.

It is entirely possible even right here, even right now.

It's fun.

THE SCAVENGING SKILL SET

To casual observers, scavenging looks easy. Gross, to some, but easy. The reasoning goes: Who scavenges? The lazy and the desperate dirt-poor. Why? Because they lack the smarts and skills and will to do anything else. Thus scavenging must be so easy that even the slackest, stupidest, most unskilled losers in the world can do it. Otherwise, they would do something else.

Q.E.D.

Not.

Scavenging is work. Getting good stuff, getting enough good stuff often enough to call yourself a *scavenger* requires skills. Discipline. Training. Time. Like skiing or heart surgery, scavenging requires detailed, specific knowledge and a skill set. Just as with skiing and surgery, natural talent helps. But just as surgeons must study anatomy and learn to cut precisely, scavengers must learn and study, too. *Where is the good stuff? Can I get it? How?*

Looks are deceiving. Sure, some scavenging takes no effort at all. Sometimes stuff falls into your lap by utter happenstance. You're in a store, say, and—voilà—someone is handing out free samples. You walk through a park or plaza just in time to see a free concert or play about to start. Carried on the wind, a five-dollar bill blows down the sidewalk and lands at your feet. Two-for-one coupons arrive in the mail. With dumb luck, sometimes scavenging *just happens*.

But.

For scavenging to be a lifestyle or a livelihood or even a hobby, we've got a lot to learn.

This chapter explores fundamental scavenging skills and practices. You don't *have* to learn them, or learn them *all*, but any one of them will make scavenging that much easier. Why not increase your yield? But more important, these skills have benefits that extend beyond scavenging. Each one of them deepens awareness, heightens sensations, and sharpens gratitude. Sure, you will be a better scavenger. You will also be more alive.

The skills mentioned below specifically apply to the category of scavenger that we dubbed "Finder" in the previous chapter. This is not really a specialized type of scavenger unto itself, but is rather just a shorthand way to describe the all-purpose full-time scavenger, those among us for whom scavenging is not merely a hobby or even a lifestyle but rather a permanent personality trait that cannot be turned off.

Want to make the jump from dabbler to maven? Want to become one with scavenging? This is what you need.

ETERNAL VIGILANCE

First: Keep your eyes peeled.

Whatever modalities of scavenging appeal to you, whatever you seek or how often or where or when, the skill you must perfect above all others is vigilance. This is because one of the few things we can say for certain about scavengeables is that they are almost always hiding in plain sight. If you liked playing Find the Hidden Pictures as a child—spying the cat, the coffee cup, and George Washington's profile in the complicated sketch of grazing cattle—you have a head start in scavenging. For us, life itself is a never-ending game of Find the Hidden Pictures.

Scavengeables almost never appear in obvious places—the sorts of venues where stuff is normally acquired. They are not usually in stores—at least not mainstream stores whose merchandise is shelved, priced, advertised, and clearly marked. No one goes door-to-door purveying scavengeables. In general, nothing and no one will point your way to scavengeables. You're on your own. Scavengeables are on the sidewalk and the ground, easy to step on or step over without a spare glance: lost jewelry, fallen cash. Scavengeables are mingled with trash. Scavengeables are literally invisible, but the wary spy subtle clues to their whereabouts: the announcement of an art opening, the hyperlink, the two-for-one coupon. Sure, some scavengeables bear FREE signs. Some await in boxes marked FREE. But even then, you have to spot the stuff, the signs, the boxes whose contours are camouflaged against hedges, sidewalks, street signs, and curbs. Vigilance comes in ever-sharpening degrees: from awake to aware to alert to attentive to all-seeing to the power to survey scenery near and far and in between, illuminated naturally or artificially or not at all, still or at any speed. After enough practice, it becomes second nature. You no longer have a semifocused setting. Your gauge is stuck on surveillance. Spacing out is not an option. Master scavengers maintain a multifocal and multidimensional hyper-omnivigilance by which they see what is as well as *what might be*. The best among us sleep with eyes half open.

The more you see, the more you get.

And we were meant to see more. Vigilance is a primal survival skill that *Homo sapiens* is built to have. Most sighted people take their eyes for granted, using vision merely as a means to get from here to there and entertain themselves. Becoming vigilant helps us become more fully realized, better in touch with our bodies.

We were so thirsty that day. It was October, Indian summer. The sun baked our hair. We never carry water bottles. We dislike the weight. Had we been downtown, we would not have *bought* a drink but might have slipped into the library, whose fountain water is ice cold. We might have visited the hardware store, which keeps a coffeepot going for customers all day. We *would* have, but we were far from downtown—crossing a residential hillside on foot with no businesses on either side for miles.

Going up to a house and drinking from its garden hose was tempting, but it's also trespassing, so no. Just two weeks earlier, two apple trees on that block were heavy with ripe red fruit. But now not even one apple remained. You'd never even know those two were fruit trees if not for the smashed, spoiled slicks on the asphalt attracting wasps.

Be vigilant, we told each other, panting in the heat as we kept walking. *Be vigilant*. Our eyes arced back and forth, back and forth. Lighthouse beams. And then—

The faintest glint. You would never have caught it, were you not primed to catch *everything*. It was obscured by leaves, but then those leaves were dead giveaways, too.

We know what grape leaves look like on the vine. Do you?

The vine clung to the outside of a garden fence, like an arm slung over the back of a couch. It was late in the season for grapes, too. These were the size of peas, half raisin. Clinging fast to the vines, they spat sticky ruby juice on our fingers as we picked them.

Juice. So sweet it pricked our eyes.

Successful scavengers are vigilant.

Try this experiment: Choose a distance to walk—one block, say, or across a park. Before taking a single step, order yourself to observe as much as you can. See how much stuff of any interest or value you can find before your short journey is over. Pretend that this has consequences—whichever would matter most to you. Pretend you are a hunter sent to feed or defend a whole clan. Pretend you are a soldier surveilling behind enemy lines. Pretend you are a tiger, an eagle, an owl—even a robot. Pretend that you will be paid for every detail you remember afterward. Pretend you are an artist seeking inspiration. Pretend you are a child.

Or pretend you are starving. Pretend you are lost. Pretend you are plotting a great escape.

Pretend your life depends on this.

Look from side to side. Look up. Look down. Most people spend their lives looking straight ahead, strictly at eye level. Their loss.

Make it a game at first. Seeing is easy. *Noticing* is hard. But once you turn it from a passive activity into an active one, once you realize how much you've been missing all your life, once you feel electrified by three words—*Look at that!*—vigilance becomes more than a game. For scavengers it is a challenge, an adventure, a link back to our ancestors who survived by scanning landscapes and surveying seas—then back even further to our ancestors who lived in trees. Vigilance is a talent you owe yourself and owe the world. Vigilance is a responsibility.

The more you see, the more you save.

What will you have gathered by the time your brief journey is over? A penny? A stepped-on toy car? A four-leaf clover? A speckled rock? A rusted 1988 DUKAKIS FOR PRESIDENT button? A crumpled-up class note from the nearby high school that says *"Look at Vanessa's shoes 2day—so UGLY!"*? The lens cap from a Nikon camera? A gold ring?

This is what life is like for the full-time scavenger. Every step you take, every time you leave your house, is a treasure hunt.

Who says you don't already have a superpower?

CURIOSITY

Get curious.

The twin sister of vigilance is curiosity. While being vigilant, you spy something: a box across the street, a glimmer on the ground. You could shrug and simply move on, thinking, *Not worth my time*, if you think anything at all. Or you could halt and wonder: What is that? Might it be something free? Something for me? Then closer. Closer. Look for clues: Is anyone around to whom it might belong? Is that a FREE sign? Closer. Are those flat things books or folded shirts? More clues: Shirts for grown-ups— or kids? Closer. Condition? Color? Cleanliness? Style? Size? Closer. Curious and close enough to touch. Aha. And is anything underneath? Is that a button? Bottle cap? Coin?

Pounce.

For most folks, curiosity is just a quirk, an extra that sometimes makes life a bit more edgy: *Josh always orders whatever looks weird on the menu!* They can turn it on or off. In fact, for standard consumers, curiosity just gets in the way.

Commercials train us at a young age to identify and demand certain brands. By 2006, American companies were spending $17 billion on ads directly aimed at children, a stratospheric increase from $100 million in 1983. Via cross-marketing, ads fill children's lives, spreading beyond TV to permeate toys and other media. Many kids' products, once purchased, themselves contain further ads for *more* products. In 2003, Procter & Gamble published *Charmin the Bear*, a beautifully illustrated book for toddlers about the adventures of the cartoon bear in its TV toilet-paper ads. A public trained to demand specific products manufactured by specific brands is a public trained to quash its native curiosity. Wondering how another product by another brand might taste or *what would happen if I went without this* is anathema. Enough such thoughts, acted upon, would smash the system. Curiosity would kill the cat *and* the capitalism. Because so much of the national economy is based on consumers doing the same things *with* the same things ad infinitum, entire industries bank on mass incuriosity, on populations who no longer wonder. And standard consumers do not realize what has been taken away from them, that this instinct is being bred out of the populace, which does and buys as it is told. In an ingenious bait-and-switch trick billions strong, consumers are *told* they are curious. They are *told* that they choose. And they want to believe it because it makes them sound lusty and alive. But stuck in their ways, wanting again and again the exact same taste or experience that advertisers have taught them to expect and that they have tasted/experienced a thousand times before—acting like addicts, terrified to stop or switch—standard consumers are curiously incurious.

Scavengers are curiously curious.

This is because we never know what we will get or where or when or even if. And if we get it, more questions arise, such as:

What is this? And, What should I do with it? And, for the philosophical among us, Why? Then comes the after-question: What will I find next?

Unbridled curiosity is mental thirst.

Every find bears a whiff of mystery that whets the curiosity that makes the finder wonder more. This feels like waking up. The find alone spurs you to wonder whose it was before, where it was bought and where it went from there and how it parted from its buyer and what it would say if it could talk.

The more you scavenge, the better you realize how much of your native curiosity has lain latent, dormant, crushed, cramped, doped into submission until now.

To coax it out and keep it sharp, try this experiment: As soon as your gaze lands on something that you do not recognize, start asking silent questions. These need not follow a narrative. Just keep pumping them out. Start with: What is that?

See how much you don't know?

The more you wonder, the harder you seek. The more you seek, the more you find.

The more you wonder, the more gifts keep giving.

TOLERANCE

Get off your high horse.

Scavenging has been reviled for centuries because it usually boils down to touching trash. Even in a retail setting, when it has been washed and sorted and priced and set out on shelves and racks, it still counts as trash. Trash that has been donated to thrift shops, carried out of homes for garage sales. Discount-outlet wares are overruns, factory rejects, damaged goods. All might be up for sale, but none are wanted by their makers or their former owners or upstanding front-run customers. Thus all are trash.

This is why we are reviled, but we know better than to revile ourselves or each other or—this matters more—to revile things that cannot help that they have been thrown out. Anyone who ever got his or her favorite chair or slip or coffeepot from a Dumpster knows better. The fact that something was thrown out has no bearing on its worth to its finder. Value is too subjective to be set by such an arbitrary state. One person's trash becomes another's treasure, zillions of times, every day. And who has the last laugh? "It doesn't have to be good to be valuable!" chortles the home page of FreeBay Cyprus, a network devoted to sharing free stuff on that Mediterranean island. Successful scavengers are not squeamish. Successful scavengers are not ashamed.

And scavengers are tolerant. To some extent we have to be, because every act of scavenging is a step out of safe, clean, stream-lined, systematic social acceptability. Every act of scavenging renders the scavenger an outsider, which helps us empathize with other types of fringe dweller. When we acquire scavengeables, it is virtually never in the standard want/get/pay/thank-you-have-a-nice-day circumstances but some alternate circumstance in which we are taking what has not been proffered, taking what is simply *there*, taking what to all appearances are other people's former belongings. Thus we must overcome our gut reflexes, our sense of danger and misbehavior, those imaginary angry-mommy slaps on our hands and angry-mommy voices in our heads hissing *Don't steal*, because we are not stealing, and hissing *Don't touch that, it's dirty*, because, yes, it might be dirty, but it won't kill me and I want it and I'm all grown up now. Most scavengeables are not perfect when we find them. They sometimes *are* dirty, just as Mommy warned, and they're dented or bent or scraped or punctured or faded or worn or past their sell-by dates. So we must overcome yet another set of gut reflexes, the age-old terror of contagion, once legitimate but now largely unwarranted in an era of high-tech sanitation. *I can wash this, and I can wash myself after carrying it home.* But until that washing, we must tolerate the presence of this unclean, damaged thing in our hands, pockets, purses, backpacks, cars.

Our levels of tolerance are intensely personal and infinitely protean. With experience, we evolve. Scavenging venues and types of scavengeables span a wide spectrum, with each point along the spectrum representing a relative degree of acceptability and a relative degree of "ick factor." For each of us, the spectrum looks different. One scavenger might avidly scavenge clothes, books, and electric appliances from everywhere except landfills and Dumpsters, but only selectively scavenge household items (rugs and towels, say, but never cosmetics or sheets)—and draw the line at everything else. Another scavenger might also avidly scavenge books, but only at library sales, and might additionally scavenge clothes, children's toys, computer components, and food, but in the former case only as hand-me-downs from friends and in the latter case only canned goods long before their sell-by dates. Yet another scavenger will take, wear, and eat anything, from anywhere. We might call this type SWL, scavengers-without-limits.

Our individual versions of the spectrum reflect our personalities, our pasts, our superstitions, our fears, and the degree to which we care about social approval. But as a rule, the more intimate or internal our interaction with the venue or the scavengeables, the greater the potential ick factor. The more visibly dirty a venue is and the more we have to exert ourselves—dig, sift, lift—the greater the ick factor. The more classifiable as trash a venue or an item is—say, a trash can, on trash day, set out for the trash collector—the greater the ick factor. The more contact an item has with our bare skin (and which bare skin on which body parts), and with our mucous membranes and/or internal organs, the greater the ick factor. Each ick factor represents a higher stratum of tolerance. With each stratum, as we acclimate ourselves to more and different forms of scavenging, we are battling and then transcending impulses and instincts that have guided our actions and the actions of everyone we know for almost as long as we can remember.

Tolerance is hard work. But remember: The more you can bear, the more you get.

BRAVERY

In a crowded, class-conscious, and gossipy society, scavenging in public and/or stating freely that you scavenge is an act of courage. The more trash you touch and admit touching—if you are not homeless or desperate but clearly doing this by choice—the braver you become.

Many standard consumers would never set foot in secondhand shops. They shudder at the very thought even of wearing what others have worn before. They gag at the idea of using silverware that entered others' mouths, even though it has been boiled and power-washed. Cold on a winter day downtown, wanting a wrap, nine out of ten standard consumers would walk past the thrift shop in order to buy a sweater or coat in the brand-new retail store for six or seven times the price. In such emergencies, suggesting the Goodwill store as a respite stocked with those urgently needed extra sweaters, coats, caps, sun hats, suitcases, blankets, or neckties to standard consumers, we have witnessed the gag. We might as well have suggested a porn shop.

OVERCOMING that old animus and outdated germ fear is a crucial skill for scavengers. Many of us feel "vibes" issuing from found stuff. Many of us have gotten "the creeps" from certain items, but this almost always has nothing to do with how dirty or clean the items are or the ambience in which we found them. If our creeps are genuine, they derive from the past history of the objects themselves, from their former owners, not from the fact that the objects happen to be lying in dumps rather than department stores. Standard consumers need never be open-minded because they inhabit controlled atmospheres. They can *say* they are tolerant, but actions speak louder than words. Successful scavengers attain a cool, collected tolerance that would impress Zen monks. Successful scavengers learn to abide deeper and deeper levels of what others would call gross. We walk the walk, not to the point of puking or infection, obviously, but enough to broaden our horizons, maximize our chances, discern glory in detritus, and make rescues.

To walk that walk, try what psychologists call systematic desensitization therapy. Also known as exposure therapy, it is a popular treatment for phobias and post-traumatic stress disorder, in which the client faces slightly escalating versions of the source of his or her anxiety. Called a "Method of Factors," the series of steps is outlined in advance, but each step is attempted only when it appears that the client is able to endure it without spinning into a breakdown. For someone with a fear of open spaces, the steps might include driving to the edge of a field, then—an hour, day, week, or month later, or however long it takes—getting out of the car and standing at the edge. Then stepping into the field, perhaps with a friend, phone, food and water, soothing music. Farther and farther into the field, with fewer and fewer accessories. The final step would be crossing the field at midday or midnight—whichever one of them is scarier—alone. A scavenging Method of Factors would start with visits to discount outlets, then to thrift stores: first with others, then alone; first to browse, then to buy. The next steps would include yard sales in upper-crust and then more ramshackle neighborhoods, then on to Dumpsters, and dumps.

Successful scavengers are tolerant but tough as nails.

TOPSY-TURVY AESTHETICS

Some scavenged objects were made to be displayed. Others were not, but their finders display them anyway. Scavenging objects that either were designed to be aesthetic or are destined to be displayed as such carries a strange responsibility. Choosing to display them privileges found objects, rewards them, honors them, and praises them. Sometimes this choice is easy. Automatic. Say you find something designed to be beautiful that actually, objectively, is. Or say you find something designed to be beautiful whose beauty is subjective, but it still appeals to you. Then you are lucky. Never does a scavenger feel luckier. Never do finds feel more like gifts. In a paved-over world, finding beautiful things is a rare and otherworldly glory. Finding an earring on the street is prospecting for gems, silver, and gold. That old manila folder in the thrown-out desk that turns out to be stuffed with lithographs is your inheritance, vouchsafed to you and you alone by someone not your kin: an accidental legacy, or somehow meant to be.

But sometimes you find something you wish you'd never seen in the first place. One day a framed painting was leaning against a stop sign with its back to us, so walking toward it, we thought, *Painting!* Paintings are always fun to find, because real human beings made them. Each is unique, not mass-produced. But poignant, because where is the painter now? Who props art against stop signs on side streets and walks away?

We both reached for it at the same time and turned it around.

It was—not good. Someone had sketched then painted an anthropomorphic cartoon tugboat with a smiling human face on its smokestack and puffs of smoke coming out. The wake was going in the wrong direction. Pencil lines showed through the paint.

Oh no, said one of us. Then tucked it under one arm, carried it across town, and brought it home.

It hung over the fireplace for two years.

Why? some might ask. Here's why: Because once you find something, in an instant you become its guardian, its parent. Whatever it is you've found, you suddenly feel empathy for it.

You think: Someone conceived this. Someone made this. Maybe a whole series of someones admired this. Poured heart and soul into this hot-pink driftwood lamp, this truck-shaped Kleenex dispenser, this amateurish painting of a cartoon tugboat. You might never normally have chosen this object or liked it one bit, but finding it instantly obligates you. Now you are its arbiter. Its judge. Or its killer, if not taking it means that no one else will, and that this object will thereby never be displayed again.

Or its redeemer. Savior. Hang it above the fireplace, even if only out of pity.

See? Successful scavengers are merciful.

BE SCAVENGING

Successful scavengers have perfected other skills and attributes as well. Patience, for instance. Ours is a waiting game. Persistence too. Composure under duress. Do not call attention to finds or to yourself as you approach. Avoid flamboyantly seizing them when others are near who might compete. Maintain a poker face. We are gamblers, too. Successful scavengers are deadpan.

And spontaneous. Say you are en route somewhere when you spy a yard-sale sign pointing the other way. Or say you were planning a quiet night at home but just found out about a clothing-swap evening organized by your sister-in-law. Successful scavengers change plans.

Successful scavengers are subtle and somewhat invisible. Successful scavengers can vanish into crowds. Successful scavengers wear clothes with nice big pockets.

LET'S SAY you have adopted some of these skills. Let's say you practiced being vigilant. And tolerant. And tough.

You'll come to realize, as do all master scavengers, that the payoff is not just finding stuff, but learning things.

Why bother becoming a scavenger?

That's why.

CHAPTER 8

THE ACCIDENTAL TAOIST

The Spirituality of Scavenging

I WENT TO SYNAGOGUE ONE DAY WITH MY TWO devout friends from out of town. They wanted to. I seldom go. That day, as always, reciting the prayers my ancestors recited, I felt nothing. Then, because I wanted to feel something, I felt guilt. Because my friends don't drive on Saturdays, we set off toward home afterward on foot. Under a hot sun in my stiff but scavenged dress-up clothes—the teal-blue rayon FREE-box top and black Z. Cavaricci trousers found ripped in a FREE box but now patched invisibly from underneath— I burned with shame as always for having felt nothing. Am I dead inside, I thought, or what? The same realization came to me that had come fifty zillion times before: *If God exists, He saw me faking it in His house.*

My friends discussed the service as we walked across a park. Clouds scudded past and, in the trees ringing the lawn, sycamore leaves rustled. My friends spoke in earnest. It had meant a lot to them and I was glad. But envious. *They have faith,* I thought. *They have something to believe in. I—*

Just then, a sparkle in the green grass caught my eye. I stooped and found a big, smooth amethyst. It filled my palm. It could not have arrived there by natural means. Raw amethysts do not occur in Northern California soil and nowhere in the mown lawns of suburban parks. And this one was not raw. It had been polished to a high shine in a tumbler, as if to announce: *Here is a gem.*

Why there, why me, why then?

Some finds feel like signals. Like signs. And like replies.

SCAVENGING TAKES US close to God.

Or *something*.

Call it God or fate or Fortean phenomena. Is there an Our Lady of Scavenging? Scavenging jolts us out of the straight, smooth, streamlined world into another where wonders manifest in gutters and hunches come true. This separate world looks like the ordinary world. This world exists within the ordinary world. We enter through the ordinary world into our world of chaos, uncertainty, and surprise. In our world, finds feel like signals and signs. Like benefaction. Benediction. Divination. Questions answered. Secrets told. In our world, turning any corner can change everything. In our world, awe strikes when we murmur, *Look at that*. To us, finds feel like gifts and dispatches from someone, somewhere, who somehow knows all about us.

Scavenging is a calling, a vocation, and a vow. Just as when nuns and monks take vows of silence, scavengers take vows of vigilance. We take vows of contentment. We take vows of tolerance. We vow never to choose. We vow to almost never spend. We vow to never be seduced by marketing. To scavengers, these are all matters of the soul.

This is true for all kinds of scavengers. Especially for finders, yes, because more than the rest of us they are truly committed to the random: finding whatever they find but never seeking it. And full-time scavengers, whose entire lives are spent outside the comforts of consumer culture, are inclined to think of matters of the soul. But even part-time scavengers, even specialized scavengers, even on-again-off-again coupon clippers, know the buzz, the transubstantiation, of *the find*.

You're sitting, standing, walking, riding, and—

Out of nowhere. Or so it seems. *The find.*

And even part-time scavengers harken to this sensation, which consumer culture with its processed, paved-over predictability has tried its best to take from us: the otherworldly, transcendental, epiphanic glory of the find.

In this processed, paved-over world, the find is the closest we come to revelations.

Proclamations. Presentations. Just for us. Some scavengers dismiss the ethereal side of our lifestyle, which is their right. The rest of us—

Commit ourselves to never knowing. Trusting fate.

Trusting fate is another phrase for faith.

This is the land of never-knowing. Scavengers live close to God—or whatever—because we live with such uncertainty. The one thing we know for sure is that we will never know. Like hermit saints or wandering sadhus, we never know what we will get or when or how or if. Like mystics, we wonder: Is this happenstance? We are washed in the magic of the random.

Most human pursuits entail at least some certainty. Only a few—gambling, say, and fishing—are as unpredictable as scavenging. In all three, you can raise the chances of success by honing certain skills, by being vigilant and patient. But your bursts of joy will always be divided by long empty spans spent waiting, watching, wondering. And when things go right, we wonder: Why this, why now, and why me? Alone against the universe when suddenly stricken with luck, we whip around looking for rivals, snares, or strings attached. Seeing none, we take what we are granted.

The land of never-knowing gives us reason to believe.

Here in the land of never-knowing, wishes condense into prayers.

WE SURRENDER

Because they can control what they consume, standard consumers believe they control their lives. At the first glint of desire, they know they can satiate it soon. They know how, with what, where, and when. Choosing their source of sweet relief in stores or at their keyboards, paying not with cash but by means abstract and symbolic—credit cards comprise magic words, magic numbers, magnetism—they feel like shamans, high priests, hierophants. Gratified instantly, some even believe they are gods. (The system wants them to.) Scavengers feel like gods sometimes, but only when finds turn us into arbiters. Normally we make no such assumptions, harbor no such hubris. We are infinitely humble, as we must be. We wear trash. We never forget how small we are in the universe.

We submit. We surrender.

Standard consumers occupy a remarkably artificial habitat, constructed for their benefit. Its every aspect is disconnected from the actualities of nature; its timetables, temperatures, sensations, stimuli, the range and number and availability of products in that habitat bear no relation to the brisk realities of nature.

Meanwhile, we scavengers keep rhythm with nature, because scavenging, like the forces of nature—storms, seas, seasons, shifting sands—is unpredictable, an ever-changing ebb and flow of dearth and bounty, speed and languor, hot and cold. Ours is life-in-the-wild, even if we seldom step outdoors.

We sacrifice. Standard consumers say, in voices slick with shock, that they could (and would) never live the way we do. *Why,* they ask, *would I want to feel deprived?* When we say we feel fine, they don't believe us. When we say our rewards are manifold, their eyebrows rise. When we say these rewards are blessings, they shiver and walk away. We sacrifice certainty. We sacrifice having stuff. The more we sacrifice, the better we know the difference between have and have-not, and the more we relish what comes when it comes. As the old Spanish proverb goes: *A buen hambre no falta salsa:* Hunger is the best sauce. Here in the land of never-knowing, we sacrifice instant gratification for the ecstasy of discovery. Here in the land of never-knowing, we sacrifice control for surprise. Here in the land of never-knowing, we sacrifice instant pleasure for the glow of gratitude. Here in the land of never-knowing, we sacrifice ease for the hard work of hope. Here in the land of never-knowing, sacrifice confirms our vows.

For us, forfeiture feels like freedom.

In a quick-fix world, taking whatever comes is holy. Walking down the street without buying a Frappuccino is a sacred act.

SCAVENGERS CAN IDENTIFY with all those who live in the land of never-knowing. We share the orisons of gamblers and fisherfolk, seeking protection, mercy, grace, but *our* kind of grace: finding stuff. At the start of the herring season every fall in the town of Clovelly on England's Devon coast, fishermen attend a special church service, reciting in unison the Clovelly Fishermen's

Prayer. Replace a few words here and there, excise references to a specific deity if you wish, and it captures what many of us feel when setting out to search, whether we say it or know it or not:

Almighty and loving Father, Thou rules in Heaven, in the earth, in the sea, and in all the deep places; there is no creature but hears, understands, and obeys thy voice. Thou speakest the word and there ariseth the stormy wind and tempest. Again Thou speakest the word and there follows a great calm. And be Thou pleased to speak a word of mercy and comfort to thy servants in their honest calling; still the winds, smooth the waves; and let them go forth and come in safety. Protect their persons, secure their vessels, and all that appertaining unto them; and let not a hair of any man's head perish. They may with Thy Disciples fish day and night and catch nothing; but if Thou pleasest to speak such a word as Thou didst then, they shall encompass so great a multitude as neither their nets nor vessels shall contain. . . . Only we beseech Thee let not our sins withhold good things from us, and therefore pardon our sins of whatsoever kind, especially our murmurings and our presumings . . . our covetousness and unthankfulness, our intemperance and our hatred, and variance with each other. . . . Thou canst by one word speaking send all these blessings to another shore, and to another people that shall serve Thee better and be more thankful than we have been. Make us Gracious Lord to consider the utter uncertainty of all our lives, and how easy it is for Thee, O Mighty God, to raise a blast, or commission a wave, and dash us against a rock. . . . Amen.

ANCIENT ROMANS worshipped Fortuna, the goddess of luck. Knowing life as a capricious dance with danger, they implored her to grant them fortune. Her temples stood all over the Roman Empire; the massive one at Praeneste, now known as Palestrina, some twenty-two miles east of Rome itself, was as big as an entire city. All of modern-day Palestrina's combined houses, schools, parks, museums, stores, businesses, and churches sit comfortably within the ancient temple boundaries. So powerful was Fortuna—whose symbols included the cornucopia, the ship's rudder, and the wheel, the precursor of today's Wheel of Fortune—that both of the major deities Jupiter and Juno were often depicted sitting on her lap, suckling at her breasts. At her festivals, fortunes were told via messages inscribed on wooden slats drawn at random. Fortuna resurfaces again and again through the centuries in literature—which proves, depending on your belief, either her true power or a human compulsion to better our chances via divine intervention. A poem in the early-thirteenth-century collection now known as the *Carmina Burana*, written by clergy in a Bavarian abbey, addresses her: "O Fortuna, / like the moon / you are constantly changing, / . . . monstrous / and empty, / you whirling wheel." She has since morphed into the inchoate Lady Luck, invoked in jest and in earnest (often disguised as jest) by gamblers, prospectors, and scavengers alike.

Even the most planned-ahead scavenging—picking plums from a well-known sidewalk tree at the height of plum season, say, or shopping for white shirts in the white-shirt section of your favorite thrift shop—has an air of uncertainty about it, a faint promise of surprise. What if all the white shirts in the shop are way too big for you or way too small? You buy some anyway and wear them anyway, and voilà: your new look. Or what if someone beat you to the tree and took all the low-hanging fruit? You research other trees—or climb. No matter how you get them, even if you pay for them, all scavenged goods—by virtue of not being new or sold full-price—can be described as finds. And finds, as such, yield an experience like no other on earth. The surprise factor, even for a heartbeat, jolts you into the spin of the infinite. The surprise factor is what children get when they find four-leaf clovers and when Daddy reappears from behind his hands, cooing *Peekaboo*.

In synagogues, I feel nothing, then guilt. Not bitterness, not angst—nothing at all. I *am* Jewish, genetically and culturally if not spiritually. Yet I am not aspiritual. I am not made of wood. Nor am I totally incapable of awe. In synagogues, I try to feel swept up, I really do, in those first-person-singular declaratives about the Infinite, the rise and fall encoded in my bones. I try. I really try. Of all the places in the world in which one should not be a charlatan, a synagogue rates high. I fidget, daydreaming of the *oneg Shabbat*, the food and wine following services. Of all those hours that I have spent in synagogues, what resonates most in my memory is the *oneg Shabbat*. Torah readings and sermons left no imprint. But those brownies, almond tarts, and tiny cups of wine. Those tuna finger sandwiches on marbled rye. Those cookies cut into Stars of David, spangled with sugar the same sky-blue as on Israel's flag. Those candied nuts. That sherbet punch. They shine in my mind decades hence like gems once glimpsed, meaning more to me than the people or the prayers. I know now that this is because they were not just sweet but free.

But synagogues per se, the refuge of my ancestors, fill me with apathy.

Catholic churches do not. I dart into them, never during Mass but when almost no one else is there. I sit staring at the statuary in the throb of candlelight, the stained-glass scenery and sculpted saints. You cannot keep me from cathedrals.

But—

I am not now and never have been Catholic. Jesus is not my personal savior and quite likely never will be.

Of course this makes me feel guilty too. Not only does my euphoria seem an insult to my ancestors—*Young lady, that's a crucifix!*—it also feels like theft, a kind of secret siphoning, a larceny not physical but spiritual because it is not the precepts and personages that these objects represent that I revere.

It is the *objects* themselves.

Yes, I worship graven images.

THE MANA OF SCAVENGING

To certain scavengers, objects are messengers: from other places, other times and lives. Each object transmits memories and history. This ennobles the object, imbuing it with a kind of soul. This is as true of staplers as of scepters. Sometimes this soul is just theoretical, in that the object makes us wonder, makes us think, makes us compassionate, connects us with humanity, and makes us thankful, which is holy. But sometimes the souls in scavenged things seem real: we find something, touch it or try it on and feel unmistakable "vibes." This is the very reason many people never scavenge: because the idea of vibes left in stuff from past owners creeps them out. And sometimes even veterans wonder whether by wearing these clothes or cooking with these pots we might somehow be taking on the fortunes of their former owners, imbibing a curse—as in Robert Louis Stevenson's "The Bottle Imp." In the story, a poor Hawaiian buys from a stranger "a round-bellied bottle with a long neck; the glass of it was white like milk, with changing rainbow colours in the grain. Within-sides something obscurely moved, like a shadow and a fire." Its glass is unbreakable because, the stranger says, "it was tempered in the flames of hell. An imp lives in it, and that is the shadow we behold there moving; or so I suppose. If any man buy this bottle the imp is at his command; all that he desires—love, fame, money, houses . . . all are his at the word uttered. Napoleon had this bottle, and by it he grew to be the king of the world; but he sold it at the last, and fell. Captain Cook had this bottle, and by it he found his way to so many islands." But the curse of the bottle is that each successive owner must sell it for less than it was bought for.

"It cannot be sold at all," the stranger explains, "unless sold at a loss. If you sell it for as much as you paid for it, back it comes to you again like a homing pigeon. It follows that the price has kept falling in these centuries, and the bottle is now remarkably cheap." Unable to imagine why anyone would ever want to sell such a marvelous thing, the Hawaiian buys it. Great fortune ensues, but when bad luck accompanies every wish granted, he becomes desperate to get rid of it. But by that time, prices have dropped so precipitously that he is told that he can get only one cent for it. Which means that whoever buys it can't sell it at all. . . .

And so it might be with what we have scavenged. How do we know that some stranger didn't put his version of the bottle imp out on the street with a FREE sign because the curse mandated giving it away? How do we know that this dusty-rose linen shirt was not someone's "unlucky shirt," worn the night her boyfriend broke up with her and then, again, the day she lost her job? How do we know that this is not the dish from which someone ate his last meal? We tell ourselves that these objects are mere fiber and glass, inanimate, insensate. But we retain traces of the animism that made our ancestors believe that spirits and gods and demons inhabited trees and rocks and talismans. Our ancestors believed in lucky charms. It has always been hard for we the living to accept that not everything is, in some way or another, living as well. Polynesian culture holds that mana, a magical force, inhabits inanimate objects. And sure enough, many of us have felt a certain happy warmth when we find certain items—and a sense of inexplicable fear or dread when we find others, no matter how dirty or clean they are, no matter how apparently unsentimental, and no matter their inherent value. They feel somehow forbidden, tainted, cursed. Just last month I found a fourteen-karat-gold chain in a flowerbed between a sidewalk and a curb. Its clasp and loop, often broken in found chains, were intact. Slipping it into my pocket, I felt that sudden lurch, a warning flutter, that accompanies about one out of every two hundred finds. I am not psychic. I cannot read palms. But something about these items says *Put it back exactly where you found it and walk on.* I always do, too superstitious to risk finding out what happens if through greed or stubbornness I were to disobey. Can objects absorb joy, pain, anxiety, tragedy? The staunchly secular would scoff. But many scavengers would not.

POSSESSIONS OF THE DEAD

In nearly all human cultures since the dawn of civilization, powerful taboos surround the dead. Many of these taboos spring from the terror that the spirits of the dead, either lonely or angry or lovelorn or unaware that they are dead, will linger in familiar places—called "haunts" for good reason—and torment the living. Funeral rites address these fears. In Navajo tradition, for instance, corpses are washed and prepared for burial by close relatives not as a privilege but as a dreadful obligation, because the dead are imbued with horrific powers. As noted by anthropologists observing such ceremonies in the American Southwest during the early 1920s, every measure was taken during the burial-preparation process to avoid "contamination." They used juniper boughs to obliterate all footprints made by the relatives of the deceased, one observer wrote, "in order to conceal from the spirit the direction in which they went." After sealing the east-facing entrance of the hogan, the low, round traditional Navajo dwelling, pallbearers removed the corpse along with a few select possessions through a hole cut into the hogan's north side. And here's the key detail: Once the corpse was out and taken away to be buried, the hogan was burned with all its contents inside. In Navajo tradition, as in others, *the possessions of the dead are taboo.*

By this measure, scavengers wallow in contamination.

Sometimes we know that the former owners of items we scavenge are still alive. And sometimes we know for a fact that they have died. But often we have no way of knowing one way or the other. The idea of wearing dead people's clothes, eating off dead people's dishes, seeing through dead people's glasses, and sleeping between dead people's sheets gives some of us a creepy feeling that all the detergent and hot water in the world cannot expunge. As a result, some perform cleansing rituals. One friend tells of a vintage beaded scarf that she got at a clothing swap. "It didn't feel icky at first," she remembers with a grimace, "until I got it home. If it was something else, like a pair of jeans or whatnot, I'd probably just have thrown it out. But that scarf was so glamorous! And someone had spent ages sewing on a million little black bugle beads." She used the same ritual that she always uses for scavenged items. After sprinkling the scarf with sea salt, she set it on a pure white platter overnight during the next full moon with a white candle burning beside it. The following morning, she made broad sweeping motions over the scarf with both hands, "like I was sweeping away the ickiness. Then I held it to my face and said into it, 'You're mine now.' Right then I could feel a shift. It wasn't creepy anymore, and it *was* mine."

BUT SETTING ASIDE the possibility of spirits, objects themselves, *just as objects*, awe us.

Some would call our awe for objects shallow, callow, dumb. In point of fact it sanctifies our lives, because for some of us each object, any object, symbolizes our vocation and what we have given up to become scavengers. And every object symbolizes our own best past finds: one stands for all. In which case every object reawakens the transubstantiation of discovery and instant gratitude. And every object is a covenant: *You will find more.*

Objects are sacred in our eyes because they have survived whatever humankind has done to them, whatever nature wrought. From the wreckage, with tales to tell, they rise.

Even new objects, freshly manufactured, not yet owned, resonate for us. They are as newborns.

For some of us, every object, any object, is a sacred object. Which makes every one of our visits to the tool closet or fridge a pilgrimage.

MAKING CONNECTIONS

Scavenging is more than just a method of acquiring stuff, or a personality trait, or a way to heal the Earth. It's also a séance of sorts: a route not merely to learning about the past but also to actually communicating with the previous owner of each item, the designer, the maker. Sometimes, fixing broken found things is more than mere tedium; it can be a lesson in reverse engineering, and reverse engineering can be a near-religious experience, a communion with the guy who, fifty years ago, designed this thing. More than that: it can open a window to the accumulated genius of the generations of inventors who came before.

Kristan likes to drag home broken electronic items for this very reason. Not only to pry them apart and see what's wrong, but to understand on a physical level why they were made this way in the first place.

A few years back he found an old early-1960s hi-fi stereo receiver in a Dumpster; unable to resist, he lugged it ten blocks home. As expected, when he plugged it in and attached it to his speakers and turntable, it didn't work. The lights came on but no sound came out. So he unplugged everything, took it apart, and looked at the dysfunctional innards.

As he puts it:

Now, I am no electrician. I do not have an engineering degree. I've never worked at a stereo component store, and I have no formal training in electronics. (Or informal training, for that matter.) But I knew that this stereo must have originally worked and now didn't; something had changed, something was wrong, and I felt I ought to be able to figure out what.

So I looked. I peered. I observed. I spent minutes, then hours, following wires from one side of the cabinet through labyrinthine connections to the other. I sniffed at fuses and welds to see if they smelled burned. I took out a magnifying glass and looked for tiny scorch marks that might indicate a bad connection. I tried to grok the entirety of how this machine was designed. If I push this button, then that closes the switch over here, which then sends a signal down this wire, which connects to this mysterious metal box; from there a yellow wire goes to this light and a blue wire connects to this other button. . . .

I felt like I was having a conversation with the bespectacled hi-fi geek in the design department of a 1961 record player company. Little by little I eliminated areas and systems and wires that couldn't possibly be the problem. My ghostly mentor with thick lenses gazing over my shoulder, shaking his head in disapproval whenever I overlooked something, nodded in satisfaction whenever I grasped a subtle design point. *So that's why the fuse has to be between the capacitor and the power cord!*

After four hours of the obsessive-compulsive hands-on reverse-engineering lesson, I had narrowed the problem down to a single green primitive integrated circuit board; the flaw was to be found there, I was sure of it. Not because I knew what the flaw was, but because it simply couldn't be anywhere else. But the board looked perfectly intact; the connections seemed solid, nothing looked burned or melted. So I took out a flashlight and my strongest magnifying glass and inspected it inch by inch. And there, almost invisible, I saw it: a tiny metallic filament of what I later determined to be Christmas-tree tinsel, which had apparently fluttered through the air vent on the stereo one long-ago winter day, landed across two pathways on the board, and created a short circuit at a fatally crucial juncture. My suspicion was that the short circuit was at first only intermittent or flickering, as the tinsel was still motile. But at some point—1966? 1971? Who knows?—a combination of cigarette smoke and dust and moisture had essentially glued the tinsel in place, and the short circuit became permanent. The stereo stopped working, so it was put in a garage. And when Dad moved to the retirement condo, it went into the Dumpster.

In the end it was so simple: I took a pair of tweezers and carefully dislodged and lifted out the quarter-inch bit of sticky tinsel.

I somehow knew, even before putting the whole thing back together and plugging it back in, that I had fixed it. And I was right. I pressed the On button and glorious stereophonic high-fidelity music filled the room. And I could feel the presence of the previous owner and the manufacturer and the designer and everyone back to Michael Faraday and Alessandro Volta standing there with me, smiling.

That is the secret joy of scavenging.

IS THIS RELIGION?

Scavenging is a practice and, for some, a lifestyle; for some, a school of thought.

Is this religion?

Well—

How DO YOU define religion? As a source of values? Check. Source of hope? Check. Source of compassion? Check. Compassion in the sense that we cannot help but wonder about the former owners of the items we acquire: Who were they? What did this thing mean to them? How and why did they part with it? Was it on purpose and, if so, in anger or in apathy? Did they regret it afterward, when it was too late, because I had taken the object away? Does the fact that this object was discarded mean that someone moved away and could not, would not, did not take it along? Is it a relic of a shattered household, a shattered relationship, the symbol of dreams blown to hell? Or a relic of childhood, now outgrown? This was loved once, now not. Did someone die? Or was this object not thrown out but lost? Does someone miss it still? Scavenging binds us to a vast network of strangers as we shoulder their possessions, ponder their passions and pain. Standard consumption affords no such touchstones. Brand-new full-price items just reflect consumers back upon themselves.

Is religion a source of charity? Check, albeit mostly inadvertent. Strangers transfer souvenirs into our safekeeping without intending to, neither knowing nor caring who we are. By becoming their beneficiaries, we transform them into benefactors. We transform their loss and their waste into generosity. Thus we redeem them from themselves.

Is religion a way to heal the world? Witness: Recycle. Repurpose. Reuse.

Is religion complete surrender? Check. In a consumer culture, choosing not to choose takes courage. No two towels in your bathroom match. This is scavenger style as surrender style. Critics might call it sloth or desperation, but it is deliberate. It is commitment. It is a bargain of faith, love, trust to wear, eat, use anything that the enigmatic wisdom of the universe allots us. Okay, we say. *Thanks!* In the FREE box outside the laundromat you find a sweatshirt that says "Firemen have longer hoses." It's clean. And you're cold. You have six hours yet before you can go home. You put it on. Another day, two guys are handing out free book bags on the college campus near your job. The book bags bear the logo of the college bisexual club. You are not bi. But these are well made, and you really need a book bag. Passersby will misread and misunderstand us. We must not mind. Our calling transcends it.

Is religion an infinite mystery? Check. Finds are otherworldly gifts. But beyond what they *are* and what they *do* and how they *look*, what might they *mean*? Are finds like koans, those cryptic questions Zen masters ask their acolytes seeking enlightenment? What is the sound of one hand clapping? Can a find or a series of finds spark an epiphany? Or are they codes? *Each of these objects I've found here starts with B. Benetton shirt, bucket, Bananarama CD.* Are finds a form of divination? *Why was that plastic Nixon mask floating in the sea? Why have my last four finds all had something to do with chickens?*

Is religion a source of comfort? Check. The free coffee and cake and live band playing in a gallery where smiling faces beckon on the loneliest day of your life. The stack of books you find when you're on your way home sick, about to spend a week in bed.

Is religion a way to become humble? Check. I for one am not ashamed to pick pennies off the ground. Scavengers are not obsessed, in this narcissistic age, with our identities. Instead, we are agglomerates of countless other closets, other kitchens, other souls.

Is religion what manifests when we say thanks? Check. All objects, even those not our own, remind us to be grateful: our own best of all. A bent spoon is better than no spoon.

Any life so laced with gratitude is laced with grace.

Is RELIGION our proof that we are not alone? Well, some finds feel too good to be coincidences. They feel too perfectly primed and timed. En route to visit a sick friend, you find on the curb a framed postcard of her favorite city in the world. You give it to her and it cheers her up. One week before a wedding to which you have nothing nice to wear, a spotless raw-silk suit turns up on the two-dollar table at a rummage sale. Depressed, you stumble upon something guaranteed to make you smile. After the first few years of this you start to wonder: meaningless ... or meant to be?

My friend Megan committed suicide last year. For three years she had been seeing a married man. One day in an e-mail he asked her to stop calling him her boyfriend. *We can still be intimate,* he wrote, *just please don't use that word.* She quietly took pills. A month later, walking along a quiet residential street at dusk, tears streaming, I thought for the millionth time, *Megan, did you actually kill yourself over a broken heart?*

The sky was slate. In the last pulse of wan midwinter sunlight I saw a glint on the ground. Yes, I am always looking down. I knelt. In the crabgrass at the foot of a sidewalk liquidambar tree was a shattered tin Christmas ornament. One of the hollow kind that comes in shapes. Half was smashed to red-silver dust, half intact. What was the shape? *A heart.* A broken heart.

RANDOM OR NOT? Lessons or luck? One day while working on this very chapter, I went out, starting the two-mile walk to town. Ten minutes after setting off, I remembered that I had left at home some DVDs that were due at the library that day. To avoid paying fees, I would have to turn back. Hiking those three blocks straight uphill, I told myself not to complain. I used to complain too much and have been trying to change. I told myself: *Good thing you remembered the DVDs before it was too late.* I told myself: *This hill is steep, but how lucky that you can walk.*

I went inside, got the DVDs, then walked two miles to town and brought them to the library. My next stop was the gym, one block away. I walk this block three times a week, sometimes on the east side and sometimes on the west. No preference. Just whim. That day, I picked the west. And there, in the gutter, was a ten-dollar bill.

At rush hour.

On a busy downtown block.

Random?

Or a reward for not complaining as I walked those three steep blocks?

Random?

Or a reward?

Would it have been there if I had *not* returned home to get those DVDs and instead arrived downtown fifteen minutes earlier?

Coincidence? No. Yes. No. Yes.

But yes.

THOUGH LESS NOW THAN BEFORE, scavengers are still scorned by the world at large. We are hated and feared and misunderstood. Just having this in common, our shared outcast status, makes us a secret society. Like other secret clans since days of old, scavengers share solidarity, unspoken understandings, and a code of ethics, and each of us tells our own tales of those finds that felt like mysteries, that felt like *something more* or *something meant*. Outsider status makes us involuntarily otherworldly. Diving into trash bins, clipping coupons, going days on end without spending a dollar, we dwell in another world. Sometimes we recognize each other on the street. Our eyes meet and involuntarily go up, as if to say: *Okay*.

BIBLICAL BIAS, REDUX

Whether or not scavenging is a religion in itself—you'll have to answer that question for yourself—it's a recurring theme in *other* religions, whose scripture and folklore present it as a behavior to be loathed, abided, pitied, or admired. It's a natural for liturgical discussions, because scavenging is a testing ground where poverty meets generosity and where cleanliness meets filth. Scavenging is a mystical realm in which one chooses and yet does not choose. As a metaphor or as a parable, scavenging is a holy test in which one is or is not satisfied with what one gets.

As alluded to in Chapter 3, the Bible has villainized scavenging for more than three thousand years.

In the Old Testament's Book of Leviticus, God tells the people of Israel in no uncertain terms which creatures they are allowed to eat and which they are not. The permitted creatures He calls clean; the forbidden ones he calls "abominations." The clean creatures include cloven-footed cud-chewers and, as God puts it, "everything in the water that has fins and scales." The vast list of forbidden creatures includes swine, shellfish, vultures, seagulls, buzzards, insects, and mice. Eating them is out of the question, but mere contact with their bodies is anathema, too: "Whoever touches their carcass shall be unclean until the evening, and he who carries their carcass shall wash his clothes and be unclean until the evening" (Leviticus 11:27 RSV). Moreover: "Anything upon which any of them falls when they are dead shall be unclean, whether it is an article of wood or a garment or a skin or a sack, any vessel. . . . And if any of them falls into any earthen vessel, all that is in it shall be unclean, and you shall break it" (Leviticus 11:31–33 RSV).

"Almost all of the creatures on the unclean list are scavengers," notes the Christian nutritionist David Meinz. But why would a compassionate God, whose children roam a desert where protein sources are scarce, make such distinctions? Buzzards might not be tasty, but to the hungry, meat is meat. Meinz is among many

modern scholars who say that the prohibitions in Leviticus are
presciently scientific. In biblical times, when sanitation and med-
icine were sparse and primitive, sharp observers noticed that eating certain creatures made more people sick than eating other
ones. Compared with cud chewers and scaly fish, animal scavengers are undiscriminating omnivores. "They don't hunt for their
own food," Meinz points out. "They eat the dead and decaying
matter of our environment. A catfish does that at the bottom of
a pond; lobsters and shrimp do it in the ocean. A pig will eat
anything." Scavenging animals often have specialized digestive
tracts that contain symbiotic bacteria that break down the toxins
in the rotting flesh or detritus they eat; but these bacteria and
toxins, if you're not careful, can be transmitted intact to whatever
(or whomever) consumes the scavengers.

YET THE OLD TESTAMENT urges compassion for human
scavengers. Not because human scavengers are so great, but because they necessarily are assumed to be downtrodden outcasts,
and God wants us to have compassion for the downtrodden. In
Leviticus, as we previously cited, God commands that scavengers
be invited onto farms to glean whatever grain and other produce
is left behind on the stalks, vines, trees, and ground after every
harvest. "When you reap the harvest of your land," God tells
farmers, "you shall not reap your field to its very border, neither
shall you gather the gleanings after your harvest. And you shall
not strip your vineyard bare, neither shall you gather the fallen
grapes of your vineyard; you shall leave them for the poor" (Leviticus 19:9–10 RSV). This injunction appears again in Deuteronomy: "When you reap your harvest in your field, and have
forgotten a sheaf in the field, you shall not go back to get it; it

shall be for the sojourner, the fatherless, and the widow. . . . When you beat your olive trees, you shall not go over the boughs again; it shall be for the sojourner, the fatherless, and the widow." It is an interesting kind of charity: rather than dole out goods or food or money to the poor, the rich were to let the poor come and get it themselves. This was meant to remind the rich that their ancestors were once poor, too: "You shall remember that you were a slave in the land of Egypt; therefore I command you to do this" (Deuteronomy 24:19–22 RSV).

We see this form of charity enacted in the Book of Ruth, which is the story of a poor young widow who wishes to support her destitute mother-in-law. Ruth declares: "Let me go to the field, and glean among the ears of grain." In the fields of Boaz the landowner, Ruth forages "without resting even for a moment" (Ruth 2:7 RSV). Touched by Ruth's dedication, Boaz asks God to bless her, and asks his laborers to make her gleaning a bit easier: "Let her glean even among the sheaves, and do not reproach her. And also pull out some from the bundles for her, and leave it for her to glean" (Ruth 2:15–16 RSV). Assembling "about an ephah"—a little more than a bushel—of barley, Ruth "took it up and went into the city; she showed her mother-in-law what she had gleaned" (Ruth 2:18 RSV).

Following those biblical orders, farmers have invited gleaners onto their lands ever since. The British artist Stanley Joseph Clark remembers how, in the Northamptonshire village of his boyhood, "after the harvest was taken from the fields, it was normal practice to hang a sheaf of corn on the field gate; this was to signify that you could start and glean the field; this practice had gone on for thousands of years, it is mentioned in the book of Leviticus." During World War II, young Clark "was often taken into the harvest fields, to help glean, [and] to finish up with very sore and bleeding legs where the stubble had pierced and scratched." He fondly remembers "collecting many ears of corn," and fears that his "will be one of the last generations to go gleaning in the fields."

It was not. Biblically inspired gleaning is very much alive today. Founded in 1979, the Society of St. Andrew is an ecumenical Christian nonprofit whose motto is "Gleaning America's Fields— Feeding America's Hungry." Volunteers from the society's "Gleaning Network" forage produce from farms and orchards nationwide after seasonal harvests, then deliver their gleanings to the needy. Such food would normally be left to rot in huge quantities. (One typical Illinois corn and potato farm offers SSA's volunteers 1,240 gleanable acres.) In 2001 alone, SSA distributed more than 45 million pounds of foraged fresh produce.

JESUS SYMPATHIZED with the poor. He would have empathized with scavengers. Always warning against greed and possessiveness, he urged his followers: "Stop worrying about your life—what you will eat or what you will drink . . . what you will wear. . . . Look at the birds in the sky. They don't plant or harvest or gather food into barns, and yet your heavenly Father feeds them. . . . Consider the lilies in the field and how they grow. They don't work or spin yarn, but I tell you that not even Solomon in all his splendor was clothed like one of them. Now if that is the way God clothes the grass in the field, which is alive today and thrown into an oven tomorrow, won't he clothe you much better—you who have little faith? So don't ever worry by saying, 'What are we going to eat?' or 'What are we going to drink?' or 'What are we going to wear?'" Only the unenlightened, Jesus insisted, are eager for these things (Matthew 6:25–31 ISV).

SWEET CHARITY

Nearly all of us have partaken of the world's most common form of biblically facilitated scavenging: religious organizations' thrift shops. These shops developed throughout the United States and the United Kingdom (where they are called, more pointedly, "charity shops") in the early twentieth century. The idea was to create a less humiliating alternative for the poor than free hand-outs: retail environments resembling ordinary full-price stores where customers—just like those at any department store or general store—could stroll the aisles, choose from a wide range of clean, presentable merchandise, and actually pay for it. The difference, of course, was that the merchandise was preowned and donated and sold at a fraction of its original cost. Counseled to treat customers with the utmost dignity and respect, thrift-shop clerks were mainly volunteers from religious charities such as Hadassah, the National Council of Jewish Women, and the Samaritans; some workers, such as at Salvation Army stores, were poor people themselves—former, current, and would-be customers—learning valuable work skills.

Some of the world's most visible thrift-shop chains continue to be operated by religious organizations. Deseret Industries, founded by the Mormons in 1938, now maintains dozens of shops in several Western states. The Salvation Army, a Christian church founded in London's East End in 1878, operates thousands of secondhand emporiums around the world. Saint Vincent de Paul was a seventeenth-century French priest whose pioneering charity efforts included orphanages, foundlings' homes, workhouses, and soup kitchens. Some of these institutions sound chilling to modern ears, but they were revolutionary in

Vincent's lifetime—a brutal era when poor urban orphans were commonly forced into prostitution and/or deliberately maimed and used as begging bait. The Society of St. Vincent de Paul—founded in 1833 by a Parisian student named Frédéric Ozanam, who was inspired by Vincent and who is a saint himself—now operates hundreds of stores. The largest of these in the United States is in Los Angeles. Founded in 1917, it measures an astounding 91,000 square feet.

SCAVENGING HEALS.

After my father died of a stroke unexpectedly, my mom found it hard to go on. She was lonely. She felt abandoned, left behind. She had no other kin, and was too private of a person to mourn in front of friends or invite them in.

The days were long. The nights were longer, just Mom and the TV set, which perched atop the wooden mount that Dad had designed, built, and painted black. She could not keep her mind on what was on TV. She could not read. She did not eat.

She went to Goodwill stores.

I had introduced her to them during my first summer after high school, when I started going there myself. Back then I wanted records, colored-vinyl records for my walls. She and Dad acted shocked at first, then went along and started buying stuff. Picture frames. Ethnic artifacts. Mom bought gigantic bracelets.

They still went after I moved away for college. They would tell me on the phone what they had bought. *Your father found an onyx owl.* They never went to thrift shops in our town for fear of running into anyone they knew. That would be too embarrassing, said Mom. They'd see us in there!

Right, I said, but you would see them, too.

No matter. She and Dad went to shops out of town, where they knew no one. *This week's bracelet tops 'em all.*

And then—

At first, after the funeral, she vowed to never leave the house again. She wouldn't have to, actually. Food was stockpiled in the garage, and anyway, she never ate. But still. Those sunny January days.

She dressed and told no one that she was going out, would never say where she was going, drove to the Goodwill store where they used to go.

She spoke to no one, knew no one. Muzak floated. It was an ordinary day. No one so much as glanced her way. And yet she thought, *They know.*

She felt a wave of sympathy welling up from the clothes, the racks, the chairs, the oblivious shoppers holding sweaters to themselves and staring into mirrors. Every shirt and dress on every rack, every shoe, every dish, carried a past, a history, and in that swirl of other places, other eras, other lives was unspeakable tragedy, and company.

She thought, *Those who do not understand will never understand.*

CRUSOE PONDERS PROVIDENCE

The all-time classic scavenging novel, Daniel Defoe's *Robinson Crusoe*, is a deeply religious book. As the sole survivor of a shipwreck, climbing ashore on an apparently uninhabited island from which he has little hope of ever being rescued, the sailor Crusoe sees his fate through a screen of Puritan values. Wondering which of his sins God is punishing him for by marooning him on this "island of despair," Crusoe veers between gratitude and agony and faith and angst. Looking back at his arrival on the island from many years hence, he muses: "I had a dismal prospect of my condition. I had great reason to consider it as a determination of Heaven, that in this desolate place, and in this desolate manner, I should end my life. The tears would run plentifully down my face when I made these reflections; and sometimes I would expostulate with myself why Providence should thus completely ruin its creatures, and render them so absolutely miserable; so abandoned without help."

Yet Crusoe had to admit that the island was not really so desolate, with its abundance of edible plants and animals and building materials. Moreover, he had made several trips back and forth to the wrecked ship, where by rifling its cabins and "rummaging the chests" he was able to scavenge several raftloads of goods, including clothes, food, weapons, ammunition, tools, navigational instruments, writing materials, and books. Along with the island's natural resources, these gleanings allowed the castaway to erect a formidable fortress of a shelter whose furnishings he built himself, again using scavenged materials and scavenged skills: "I had never handled a tool in my life; and yet, in time, by labor, application, and contrivance, I found, at last, that I wanted nothing but I could have made it . . . I made an abundance of things." His successful scavenging had taught him a lot, and it made him more optimistic. "It occurred to me . . . how well I was furnished for my subsistence," he admits. Lucky, too, was he to have survived the wreck, and lucky that the ship had stayed afloat so long "that I had time to get all these things out of her." Crusoe reflects at length on this, exulting that "the good providence of God . . . wonderfully ordered the ship to be cast up near to the shore, where I not only could come at her, but could bring what I got out of her to the shore, for my relief and comfort."

Newly confident, Crusoe sat down to his island meals "with thankfulness, and admired God's providence, which had thus spread my table in the wilderness: I learned to look more on the bright side," he confides. What a far cry this scavenger was from "those discontented people ... who cannot enjoy comfortably what God has given them, because they see and covet something that he has not given them. All our discontents about what we want, appeared to me to spring from the want of thankfulness for what we have." Three hundred years later, no present-day scavenger could say it better.

WORLD RELIGIONS

This Sufi tale, translated by Idries Shah, is as many as a thousand years old:

"A scavenger, walking down the street of the perfume-sellers, fell down as if dead. People tried to revive him with sweet odours, but he only became worse. Finally a former scavenger came along, and recognized the situation. He held something filthy under the man's nose and he immediately revived, calling out: 'This is indeed perfume!'"

At first this sounds like a joke. A closer look reveals these scavengers as enlightened and wise. Perhaps the fancy potions symbolize the shallow surface niceties of life and "something filthy" symbolizes authenticity. Unmoved by fancy potions, scavengers respond only to raw reality. Filth keeps us real.

THE FIRST of Buddhism's Four Noble Truths is that all life is suffering. The second is that suffering is caused by desire. As

Gautama Buddha defined it after emerging from his epiphanic meditation under the Bodhi Tree, desire is a yen for pleasure, possessions, and youth.

In other words, desire means *want-get.*

Desire, said Gautama Buddha, makes us greedy, envious, and bitter and keeps us from finding inner peace.

Consumerism is desire.

Also known as Shakyamuni and as Siddhartha and by various other names, Gautama Buddha was born into a noble family in the sixth century BCE in what is now Nepal. Raised entirely within the walls of a palatial compound, the teenage Gautama happened one day in the palace gardens to see a doddering white-haired old man. Soon afterward, he saw a corpse being borne on a bier, surrounded by mourning relatives. Having been cut off from the real world all his life, Gautama was appalled to see the ravages of age and death. The depths of human suffering—and the idea that the more we love, the more we suffer when we lose it—struck him to the core. Going against his father's wishes, leaving behind his sixteen-year-old wife, Yasodhara, Gautama strode out into the world vowing to study with sages and learn the meaning of pain.

Early in his sojourn, still dressed as a prince, he met a poor hermit with whom he offered to trade clothes. The hermit went off happily in princely castoffs. Gautama went off determinedly in the traditional begging robe made of patchwork scraps known, in Sanskrit, as *pāmsūda.* Historic texts setting specific parameters for *pāmsūda* reveal what Gautama's robe was made of. The scraps could be of cloth that had been burned by fire, chewed by oxen, gnawed by mice, or worn by the dead. Furthermore, the scraps were to have been scavenged from trash heaps, from the fields, from roadsides, or even from cremation grounds. As much of each piece that could possibly be reused was washed, cut into rectangles, fashioned into a robe, and tinted with plant dye to create the earthy tone traditional for beggars' garb, and called, in Sanskrit, *kashaya*. For food, Gautama begged door-to-door and scavenged edible grasses, moss, and—mortifying himself as ascetics do—cow dung. He augmented his costume by scavenging bark, leaves, and bits of carcasses: fur, feathers, tails. Under the now renowned Bodhi Tree—a majestic fig located in what is now the Indian state of Bihar—Gautama had a series of revelations known as the Noble Truths. He taught these to an ever-increasing clamor of followers, setting in motion an anticonsumerist, antimaterialist creed that spread around the world.

Buddhists believe that desire causes suffering. They define desire as attachment, yearning, and possessiveness. They believe that we can reduce desire and break its cycle if we savor every moment, every breath and blink. Scavengers are good at this: it helps us find stuff. So we inadvertently excel at a key Buddhist skill. The fact that we seek *stuff* disqualifies some of us from enlightenment. But it's a matter of degree. Those who do not seek so much as simply find—the minimalists among us—still qualify. And just by being scavengers, most of us already embrace the basic Buddhist values of simplicity, conservation, preservation, improvisation, humility. We who wear garbage cannot put on airs. In Buddhist literature and lore, these traits—*our* traits—are praised. "For incense, I placed a plum branch in a jar," explained the thirteenth-century Chinese Buddhist monk Shi Wu in one of his many poems celebrating life as a hermit. "On snow-filled nights, a fire is my companion."

Scholars say Buddhist values turned recycling into standard practice during Japan's two-plus centuries of isolation from the West: the Edo period, which ended with the demise of the shogunate in 1868. Secondhand shops and entire secondhand districts peppered Edo, the bustling metropolis that became Tokyo. Secondhand dealers who lacked their own shops toted used goods around town in four-legged bamboo baskets; because of the baskets, Edoites called the dealers "bamboo-horse clothing sellers." A flea market began daily at dawn. Scavengers collected broken pots and metal fittings from the ashes of house fires and resold them in a thriving scrap-metal trade; in the year 1723, a total of 793 scrap-iron shops were registered in Edo alone. Wholesalers traveled from region to region throughout Japan, buying and selling used goods of all kinds in bulk. As cotton became a common fabric in the island nation during that period, cotton clothes went from wearer to wearer until finally, unfit for wear, they were efficiently taken apart and repurposed into rags, diapers, and other useful items. It was a fact of Edo-era life that objects were to be used, reused, repurposed, and reused some more until they fell apart. Two centuries later, Western influence and mass production have turned Japan into one of the most flagrantly wasteful societies on earth. Its garbage dumps are piled with massive quantities of nearly new goods every year.

BUT JUST BY SCAVENGING—whatever faith you were born into and whatever, if any, you practice now—you are an accidental Taoist.

Practiced by some as a religion—with a pantheon of deities who judge and punish and reward—and by others as a rather secular philosophy, Taoism has roots in prehistoric China, far predating Buddhism, which it later influenced. Neither form of Taoism is strictly antimaterialistic: those scarlet wooden shelves you see mounted on walls in Chinese restaurants and other businesses, lit with red bulbs as incense burns before pictures of gods, are Taoist prosperity shrines, blatant pleas for wealth.

But the core of Taoism is an intangible force known as the Tao, which literally means "the way." Endless and boundless, the Tao comprises the ebb and flow of all existence, the *yin* and *yang*, dark and light. Its qualities, its imponderable order-within-apparent-chaos, are elucidated in the *Tao Te Ching*, a collection of cryptic epigrams whose mysterious origins date back to the third or perhaps even the sixth century BCE. Allegedly written by a wandering hermit named Lao Tzu, the *Tao Te Ching* sets out a worldview that many scavengers would feel speaks for them.

"When people see some things as beautiful," one epigram reads, "other things become ugly. When people see some things as good, other things become bad."

That's just how we feel! Trash is treasure!

"Stop wanting stuff," warns another epigram. "It keeps you from seeing what's real." As objects leap from life to life, swirling from stranger to stranger, and we wait and watch and wonder when or where and ask why, we scavengers know all about the flow. We know. Other epigrams warn against intolerance, impatience, and pointless activity: heck, straight out of the scavengers' playbook. The *Tao Te Ching* could be the veritable scavenging Scripture. A fundamental Taoist concept is *wu wei,* meaning "nonaction." This doesn't mean paralysis or weak passivity but rather patience, acceptance, a going-with-the-flow that neither looks nor feels forced. This spirit informs tai chi, kung fu, wushu, and other Chinese martial arts that appear languid and random yet require masterful balance, flexibility, and insight.

As does scavenging.

"Do what you have to do, then walk away," urges the *Tao Te Ching*. "Otherwise, you'll lose your mind."

"No crime is greater than greed," it warns. "No calamity greater than discontent, no fault worse than possessiveness. He who is contented with contentment shall always be content. . . . If you realize that you have enough, you are truly rich."

Amen.

CHAPTER 9

THE SCAVENGER CODE OF ETHICS

The Twelve Commandments of Scavenging

FREEDOM IS SCARY. BECAUSE ONCE YOU'VE FREED yourself from an oppressive environment, you realize that up until then you had been coasting on the rules and guidelines set down for you by your oppressors. Mom and Dad made you eat broccoli and enforced an eleven p.m. Saturday-night curfew. But when you finally move out on your own—then what? At first, having no rules feels like paradise. Yet after a few months of junk food and all-night parties, you realize: *I can't live like this forever. I've got to make my own rules now.* And then one evening you look down at your dinner plate and think, *What the—? I'm eating broccoli voluntarily.*

Now that the age-old prejudice against scavengers is lifting, the time has come to figure out our own moral code. We as a group need to decide for *ourselves* the standards by which scavengers should live. We need a code of ethics.

Of course, we are merely authors, not prophets on a

mountaintop, so the rules and suggestions you see here are not inviolable laws from on high but rather the starting points for a discussion. If you think something is missing from this Scavenger Code of Ethics, by all means add your own commandments, warnings, vows, protocols, and provisos.

But if you want to embrace the scavenging philosophy, try your best to follow these principles.

1. DO NOT STEAL

Scavenging is not about taking other people's stuff. It's quite the opposite: It's about acquiring things that others don't want, or have discarded, or have no use for, or simply ignore. Doing anything that might remotely be classified as theft not only is illegal, but undermines the very principles of scavenging; and by using scavenging as a cover story for theft, you ruin things for everyone else because you confirm the worst suspicions that society has about scavengers.

However, as with all seemingly straightforward commandments, this one has gray areas that can be hard to interpret. The best route under any such circumstances is to *ask*.

Is this yours?

Did you lose this?

Do you want this?

And if there's no one to ask, then go with your heart.

A real-life example: While out walking recently, we passed some seemingly haphazard piles of old furniture and other musty junk on the sidewalk of a little-used street. A quick perusal of the piles revealed several interesting tidbits that just begged to be scavenged. These included some World War I–era sheet music with humorous covers, a very old family photo album, some valuable-looking porcelain dishware. But to whom did it belong? Was it being discarded? Or was somebody just moving away? And if it *was* being discarded, had somebody already claimed it? The only way to know for sure was to ask. We spied an open garage down a driveway, called out a greeting, and a young man emerged. When asked, he explained that he was a hauler hired to empty out the garage. And that the piles were not all the same; the smallest pile was stuff he was keeping for himself. Another pile off to the side was stuff he was saving for the owner of the hauling company; but the main pile was indeed headed for the dump. And we were free to scavenge whatever we wanted from it. Which is exactly what we proceeded to do. He even reached into the pile to help us, offering a framed painting he thought we might not have seen. Had we not asked first, we might have accidentally stolen something that the hauler had claimed for himself.

2. DO NOT HARM THE ENVIRONMENT

One of the best reasons to become a scavenger is to help the Earth. So it would be counterproductive to *damage* the environment while trying to save it.

Never, ever remove living plants or animals from national parks, tide pools, or other environmentally sensitive areas.

If you are metal-detecting on bare ground, always completely refill whatever holes you dig.

If you are metal-detecting on grass, try to make a flap or plug of turf that can be replaced after you've searched underneath it, so the lawn looks undamaged and can easily heal when you're done.

After scavenging in Dumpsters, FREE boxes, or other containers, replace everything that you aren't going to take. Keep the surrounding areas tidy. Don't leave junk scattered around.

When searching through a pile of discarded material, don't draw it out over a wider space and make a big mess of it. Leave the pile essentially as neat as (or neater than) you found it.

Don't drive your SUV twenty miles to recycle one bundle of newspapers or to save two dollars on an advertised sale.

In general, consider the full eco-cost of whatever you're doing.

3. LIVE COMFORTABLY; DON'T DENY YOURSELF NECESSITIES JUST TO PROVE YOUR SCAVENGING CREDENTIALS

Scavenge only if it makes you happy or if you have no choice, but don't scavenge as a way to punish yourself.

Scavenge for fun; scavenge as a hobby; scavenge as a profession; even scavenge as a lifestyle. But scavenging can actually get dangerous when it becomes an obsession or compulsive hoarding, or when it becomes a form of self-harm or self-mortification.

If you have a fix-it/hands-on/DIY personality, one of the secret joys of scavenging is acquiring not simply decorative items or nonessential knickknacks, but functional items that you can actually *use*. For example, not long ago our telephone cord became frayed and no longer worked properly. No need to go to the store and spend ten dollars on a new cord—why, here's a perfectly good replacement cord that we found long ago and stowed away in the closet . . . *rummaging around . . . where is it, where is it* . . . here! With this principle in mind, consider saving any sort of scavenged functional object that might come in handy in the future.

The potential problem arises when you develop a need for something that you have not yet found and do not currently possess. Do you try to scavenge a replacement? Or do you just give in and buy it new at a store? There is no definitive answer; it depends on how essential the item is, how time-sensitive, and how easy it might be to scavenge.

Fairly recently I broke the sole pair of nonprescription sunglasses that I used on sunny days. Now, I know from long experience that sunglasses are a fairly common scavenged object. Not only are they often found on bus benches, in city parks, at picnic sites, and many other places where their wearers remove them and leave them behind, but in a pinch they frequently crop up at garage sales for fifty cents or less. And though I might be picky about my sunglasses, I'm not *that* picky. So after losing these, I thought: I'm sure to soon find something I like. No need to go to some overpriced optometrist and buy a seventy-dollar pair of sunglasses. And sure enough, just three days later, I found a pair of *very* nice Ray-Bans simply lying on a park lawn in San Francisco, accidentally dropped by a tourist or jogger. It was as if I had specially ordered them from the scavenging gods, who delivered a free pair exactly to my specifications.

But that was a fortunate circumstance. If I hadn't stumbled on that pair, how long should I have waited for my sunglasses to be delivered to me through serendipity? A week? Two weeks? A month? How long do I walk around squinting into the glare and getting eye strain, as I scour the sidewalk for glasses that someone else dropped? Am I mad? At what point does putting one's faith in luck turn into a form of demented self-denial?

About six months ago we found a DVD player in a FREE box, which we brought home and discovered to be perfectly functional. And not only did it work fine, it was *better* than the DVD player we already had, in that it displayed subtitles more consistently and operated more quietly. But our new find had one flaw: it lacked a remote control. Before I switched DVD players, I'd need to get a remote control for the new one, either one made by the same company or one of those universal remotes that can be programmed. I certainly had no intention of *buying* a new remote control; after all, our old DVD player still worked. This new one was merely an upgrade, not a necessity. But it wouldn't be an improvement if we had to get up and press the buttons manually each time we wanted to pause or restart or fast-forward a movie. So I added "remote control" to the long invisible list I keep in my head of items to look out for while scavenging.

Well, that was six months ago. And I *still* haven't found the right kind of remote control. Someone at a garage sale did give me a universal remote, but I think it was broken because I never could get it to work. As a consequence, our beautiful new functional DVD player still sits behind the TV, collecting dust, awaiting completion.

Notorious Gilded Age millionairess Hetty Green was one of the wealthiest women in the world during the nineteenth century, and yet she scavenged leftover scraps of soap and saved them in a tin box so that they could be molded into new bars and reused. She made her children wear scavenged clothes bought for pennies from a rag dealer. All the while, her net worth exceeded $200 million, which (depending on how you calculate it) would be worth between $4 billion and $10 billion today. There's scavenging for fun and scavenging because you care about the environment—and then there's scavenging as a symptom of some underlying pathology. Hetty Green is still famous as "the greatest miser who ever lived," and she went to unimaginable lengths to avoid spending any money at all; scavenging was only one small aspect of her lifestyle. She allowed her son's leg to be amputated rather than pay for a doctor to treat it properly; she often lived in small, dingy apartments because they were inexpensive; she conducted her business affairs in a borrowed office; she bickered with shopkeepers over the prices of the smallest items—all while accumulating what at the time was nearly incalculable wealth.

Green suffered from some undiagnosed personality disorder, and she embodied precisely the lifestyle this commandment warns against. We try to scavenge whatever we can, but there are times when we simply need to buy things new. Prescription medicines, for instance. And when our refrigerator conked out about ten years ago, we didn't prowl the streets at night to see if we could hunt down a discarded refrigerator. No. We went to the store and bought a brand-new energy-efficient model. (After seeing which ones were on sale, naturally.) Not only did we not want to live even one day without a decent refrigerator, but the truth is, most discarded fridges have been discarded for a very good reason. People tend not to throw away clean, functional refrigerators.

So, while I *will* spend a few days waiting to see if I can scavenge some sunglasses, or six months waiting for a remote control, when it comes to refrigerators and other essentials—no way. And it's this key detail that scares some people away from the scavenging lifestyle—they think they must degrade themselves or live uncomfortably for the sake of some absurd intangible principles. Just always remember that one should scavenge only up to but not beyond one's comfort level. If you're okay with scavenged food—go for it. But if the very thought nauseates you, then please, don't force yourself to eat something from a Dumpster just to prove your scavenging bona fides.

4. DON'T BECOME A NUISANCE TO YOUR SOURCES OR YOUR NEIGHBORS

Let's be honest: sometimes scavengers can be terrible neighbors. Especially the kind of scavenger who doesn't have enough room to store all the stuff he drags home. We knew a professional scavenger—let's call him "Howard"—who was the neighbor from hell. Several times a week he brought home another vanload of discards and miscellanea that he acquired during his near-daily scavenging runs. He long ago ran out of room inside his house in a slightly run-down residential neighborhood, so he began stacking up the new arrivals in his driveway. The neighbors complained at first, so Howard bought a prefab storage shed and put it in the backyard. But within a very short time the storage shed was itself overflowing, so once again the driveway began to fill up with junk.

Now, many scavengers, ourselves included, take into account an object's *size* before deciding to keep it. The smaller it is, the more open we are to bringing it home—because we know that oversize objects are a hassle to transport and even more of a hassle to store. Not so with Howard—he'd take anything, dimensions be damned. And so the piles in his driveway grew taller and wider: armchairs and car windshields and plastic swimming pools and weed eaters and tomato stakes and railroad ties and washing machines and tricycles and potted plants and deflated bouncy castles and camper shells and overhead projectors and Sheetrock and antique bathtubs and golf bags and adjustable drafting tables and redwood burls and terrariums he had accumulated from abandoned storage lockers and estate sales and Dumpsters and sidewalk giveaways. Howard was indiscriminate because scavenging was his main source of income. He brought home most of this stuff with the intention not of keeping it but rather of selling it as quickly as possible. The piles in the driveway were temporary, he told the neighbors. Not to worry; it would all be gone soon.

Unfortunately, the process of selling the stuff only served to amplify the nuisance factor, as a constant stream of junk dealers and flea marketers and craigslisters and recyclers and other characters milled around on Howard's property at every hour of the day and night, negotiating prices. Thieves, too, would show up at three in the morning and try to abscond with as much stuff as possible before the cacophony awoke Howard or his increasingly infuriated neighbors.

And despite all this, the piles did not diminish: Howard acquired stuff much faster than he could sell it, and the piles spread across his front yard and porch. Before long Howard had become what every neighbor dreads: an exhibitionist pack rat. Howard had started to become attached to some of his finds, and though they remained theoretically for sale amidst the piles, he had developed such a bond with the shortwave radio and the 1930s baby carriage and the Darth Vader costume that he demanded outrageous prices for them, knowing that no one would want to pay that much. As the months turned into years, what had begun as a temporary holding zone for his recycled junk business slowly transmogrified into what was essentially Howard's Outdoor Museum of Scavenged Treasures. Little by little all the salable items were carted off and all that remained were his prized finds, now covering nearly every square inch of his property.

Now, you might be thinking: Isn't there a law against blight? Why didn't his neighbors call the police? Well, they did. All the time. But all the police could do was give warnings and issue tickets. Because the law, as it turned out, was rather toothless, and the worst penalty Howard could be subjected to was a $500 fine.

Per year. He kept promising to clean things up, and tried to protest a couple of the fines in court, but ended up pleading penury and saying he couldn't afford to pay them. So the fines kept growing, but nothing ever changed. And the police began telling the neighbors that their crime-plagued city had higher-priority problems than a junk pile in a driveway. Would you rather we catch murderers, asked the cops, or spend our time issuing tickets for Howard's messy yard? Because we don't have time for both.

Things continued this way for years, until Howard finally injured his back on a scavenging run and no longer had the strength to bring much stuff home anymore. The extent of the mess began to decrease a bit, but even to this day Howard's yard remains a disaster, which he surveys from his porch with a mixture of indifference and avuncular pride, as if the junk were a member of the family.

Howard is the stereotypical example of why scavengers get a bad reputation: he violated Rule 4 of the Scavenger Code of Ethics and became a nuisance to his neighbors. And all it takes is a few Howards to give us all a bad name.

Don't be like Howard.

Yet there's something just as annoying as being a nuisance to your neighbors—and that's being a nuisance to your sources. Often, when a scavenger finds a person or a place that is a reliable font of scavenged stuff, the tendency is to keep coming back for more. If you do this, don't be aggressive or invasive. Because you'll risk turning off the source for everyone.

If a friend gives you his old computer because he got a new one for Christmas, and then shortly afterward also gives you his old printer because he doesn't need it anymore, don't go back to him six months later and ask if he has any more spare computers lying around. It's one thing to be the grateful recipient of a gift, and quite another to be a greedy scrounger. If someone lets you pick apples from her overabundant front-yard tree, don't break off branches or drive up with an industrial-size crate and strip the tree bare. Just take a few pieces or bagfuls of fruit and be courteous.

One of our secret sources of high-quality scavenged food was for years a chi-chi bakery that had a special bin outdoors in the back. The bin was exclusively for misbaked, day-old, and imperfect loaves of bread. No other garbage was ever allowed in the bin, and it had a sealed lid, making it rainproof, ratproof, and sanitary. A couple times a week, by arrangement, a local organic farmer would show up with a truck and empty out the bin, bringing the loaves back to feed his free-range chickens and pigs and goats. Quite an efficient setup, considering that most bakeries just throw away their discards. But many of the "imperfect" loaves that ended up in this bin were so imperceptibly imperfect that they seemed just as good as the ones in the store—better, actually, since the ones in the bin had often just emerged from the ovens and were fantastically fresh.

Now, word started getting around in the local scavenging circles about this amazing source of free gourmet fresh-baked bread—just so long as you didn't mind taking it out of a discard bin. Yet the bakery's management didn't want to get sued for providing unsanitary food. So their official policy was: No Scavenging Allowed. And if you were unlucky enough to be caught by one of the owners as you peered into the bin, he'd give you a talking-to and explain that they couldn't allow human consumption of the discards, no matter how good they smelled. But, as we learned, this was mostly just an act to cover themselves legally. The employees, who were on site 95 percent of the time, generally had no problem with scavengers snagging the occasional loaf from the bin; as the ones baking the bread, they knew it was perfectly edible, marred only by some minor cosmetic flaw. So if you knew the secret location, and knew the right time to stop by, and were okay with scavenging food, you could keep yourself supplied constantly with delicious fresh-baked bread.

And then the nuisances had to ruin it for everyone. First they'd show up and take not one or two loaves, but five or ten. Then they'd bring their friends and take twenty or thirty loaves. Then "homeless advocates" began using the bin as a primary source to supply food banks, extracting dozens of loaves every day. And if the bin was empty, some brazen bozos would knock on the bakery's back door and ask if any day-olds or misbaked loaves were arriving soon. And that was the breaking point. The owners had finally had enough.

One day not so long ago, we went by the bakery, only to find that a new fence had been built around the parking lot, and it was securely padlocked. The delivery drivers had to get out and unlock it and relock it every time they arrived or departed—but it was the only way to keep the overly aggressive scavengers out. A small sign on the fence reiterated the rule that the bread in the discard bin was NOT free for the taking. And that was the end of that.

So for the sake of your neighbors and your sources and all the other scavengers out there: Don't be a nuisance.

5. DON'T REMOVE HISTORICAL OR ARCHAEOLOGICAL ARTIFACTS FROM AREAS WHERE THEY ARE PROTECTED

The United States is full of historical sites that are protected by law. Battlefields, ghost towns, Native American settlements, archaeological sites, historic buildings, and so on. As tempting as it might be, never, ever remove any artifacts of any kind from protected sites such as these. It might *feel* like scavenging, especially when no one else is around, but there's another name for it: looting. And it's a scavenging no-no.

That doesn't mean everything antique is necessarily off-limits. If you're out metal-detecting and find a musket ball in an unmarked area or in a known battlefield where collecting artifacts is allowed, then by all means you can keep it. And not every abandoned farm counts as a "ghost town": sometimes an abandoned farm is just that—abandoned, so feel free to clean off that wagon wheel you found in the field and take it home.

We once faced a difficult moral dilemma on this very issue— scavenging archaeological artifacts. Several years ago we were traveling through Sicily doing research for an earlier book (about temples). As part of our pretrip research, we had tracked down the locations of various well-known *and* obscure Greek and Roman temples that had been built in Sicily eons ago. Many of these, when we visited, had been turned into government-run archaeological sites, where for a small fee one could tour the ruins. In some cases they were popular and crowded; but most were far off the beaten track. Sometimes we'd show up at the site of an ancient temple, only to find a modern apartment building or a freeway overpass built on the site, usually after everything of value had been extracted from the dig.

Ah, but once, at a location we can't divulge, we trekked out to find the rumored remains of one of the oldest Greek temples on Sicily, and found ourselves in a desolate area of sand dunes at dusk, within earshot of waves breaking on the shore. My notes told me that the remains of a significant temple complex (built by the Greeks when Sicily was still a Greek colony, before the Romans arrived) had been excavated here in the nineteenth century; yet nothing was visible for miles around except sand dunes and windblown weeds. After a brief and fruitless search, we sat down defeated in the sand. We had had this same experience several times on the trip already—archaeologists had excavated a site long before, removed absolutely everything, then filled in the hole and let it return to nature, as if there had never been anything there to begin with. The books we had gleaned our information from were often not modern travel guides but rather musty archaeological tomes written long ago, and there was no way to know in many cases what the "temple" looked like today.

So we rested a bit before turning around and heading back to civilization, absentmindedly trailing our fingers through the sand, when . . . *what's that?* Anneli felt something smooth and hard just inches below the surface. She worked it loose and lifted it free into the air, grains of sand trailing off: a marble sculpture fragment of a human foot, still gleaming white after 2,500 years under the dunes. Before she could even exclaim, at that same moment my finger brushed something round under the sand, and I extracted a tiny votive clay pot, just two inches in diameter, painted with wavy brownish-red lines, faded but still visible. Also quite obviously made by Greek colonists 2,500 years ago.

What words can express our emotions at that moment? It was, for me at least, a scavenger's dream come true. Better than that: something I hadn't even dared to dream. With wide eyes and cries of glee, we began digging into the sand frenetically, and the dunes gave forth their treasure: clay shards and broken pots and bits of statuary and votive lamps and corroded disks that had once been copper coins. The jointed limbs of an ancient child's doll. Every find brought more waves of excitement and speechless astonishment.

After about ten minutes I paused to reread the notes I had brought—photocopied pages from a century-old monograph about this temple complex. Toward the end I noticed a detail that I had glossed over originally: the nineteenth-century archaeologists had discovered, behind the temple itself, the "temple dump," a deep and wide pit where everything had been discarded for centuries and centuries until the complex fell into disuse. They described finding such a proliferation of broken crockery and discarded votive pots that, after carting off nearly a ton of material, they simply gave up; and having deemed the dump of no further interest, they just covered it back up without having extracted all its contents, since the broken shards they found filling the dump paled in comparison with the full-size unbroken pots and intact statues they had uncovered (and carried away) elsewhere on the site.

So the scattered bits and pieces we were sifting from the dunes were not only discarded by the original temple inhabitants, they were discarded *a second time* by the archaeologists. Surely something thrown away and unwanted *twice* was scavengeable—right?

Unfortunately, it wasn't as clear-cut as that. Because we knew full well that Italy has a national law forbidding the removal of antiquities from the country without a permit. And here we were clutching armloads of glorious, intoxicating antiquities. What to do?

We began rationalizing. Surely the law was made to stop people from chipping off parts of the Colosseum and similar well-known ruins to bring back as souvenirs. Also, Italy doesn't want people to loot heretofore undiscovered tombs and sell priceless antiquities on the black market. But these? These broken pots and bits of marble that thrilled us personally were quite worthless, archaeologically speaking—so worthless that the professionals who had excavated the site just threw them back and abandoned them. Furthermore, this was no undiscovered tomb or unknown treasure: it was already fully excavated and documented, and every bit of historical data had long ago been extracted from the site. If we were to just leave them here, what good would it do anyone? It's not like there would ever be another dig here—the site was of no further interest to archaeologists. What were we to do—just dig a hole in the sand and put everything back? What a tragedy, what a waste that would seem. Eventually it would all get exposed and eroded away by the wind, or washed out to sea at high tide, as undoubtedly countless other little bits had done over the centuries.

So much for the rationalizations. The other halves of our brains were thinking, "If we get caught with these artifacts by the border police, we're going to find ourselves in an Italian prison."

What to do? Paralyzed by our ethical dilemma, we sat out on the dunes until night had fallen, mulling our options. And we finally hit on a plan: We *were* going to take the shards and ancient garbage with us, but we *weren't* going to try to "smuggle" them out of the country surreptitiously. We wouldn't hide them at all. Because my theory was that the border guards wouldn't think they were even real to begin with.

We'd noticed that souvenir shops and tourist shops in Italy and Greece, especially near archeological sites, often sold faux antiquities and even faux shards. Furthermore, if you looked like a big enough sucker, you might be approached by a shady character offering to sell you "real" Roman or Greek artifacts that inevitably ended up being counterfeit. (We'd met a few other travelers who had fallen for the scam.) So any guard who saw our "antiquities" would laugh them off and assume they were fake anyway.

We took as much stuff as we could carry back to our hotel, and a week or so later, when we were flying out of the country, we put them in plain sight in our carry-on luggage at the airport in Rome. Through the X-ray machine—the operator didn't bat an eyelash. A customs guy then perfunctorily pawed through our bags, looked right at the bits of marble and pottery, and waved us through. And that was it—the whole thing went off without a hitch.

So why are we telling this story? Didn't we violate our own Rule 5, "Don't remove historical or archaeological artifacts from areas where they are protected"? Well, yes . . . and no. We certainly aren't *proud* of what we did. But then again, I for one am not entirely convinced that we did anything "wrong," because the rationalizations mentioned above were all true: neither the Italian government nor the archaeologists nor anyone else cared about these broken bits of ancient garbage anymore. Whom were we hurting? If anything, this incident also illustrates how we *followed* a principle stated in Rule 1: Scavenging is about "acquiring things that others don't want, or have discarded, or have no use for, or simply ignore." Think of this anecdote as food for thought: an example of the kind of moral dilemmas you as a scavenger will have to face when trying to live up to the Code of Ethics.

6. MAKE AN EFFORT TO RETURN LOST THINGS OF GREAT VALUE IF THE OWNER CAN BE FOUND

This self-evident rule of thumb applies to everybody, not just scavengers, but it has special significance to us because, well, we find more things than most people do. Scavengers are the ones with their eyes on the ground, who are scanning sidewalks and gutters and who are glancing behind museum benches and checking under their movie theater seats. We find nickels and watches and bifocals and shopping lists and baseball caps and, yes, even the occasional ten-dollar bill. In most circumstances you are free to keep such things. What else can you do, raise the ten-dollar bill above your head during downtown rush hour and yell, "Anybody lose ten bucks?"

But the thrill of finding something valuable can become a moral dilemma when the owner of that something can possibly be identified. In particular: wallets, credit cards, and cell phones. Every Boy Scout—hell, anybody with a conscience—knows that when you find a wallet, the right thing to do is try to contact the person who lost it. All you have to do is imagine how *you'd* feel if you lost *your* wallet, and the empathy gene kicks in. Returning it makes you feel good, part of the human community.

I've found and returned literally dozens of wallets in my life, but the results have often been not quite what I imagined. Recently, I've become more cynical and even felt tempted to violate my own rule. It all started when I was only six years old, and I went to the corner candy store to buy a Popsicle with my dime. (Yes, six-year-olds once did things like that, all by themselves.) I reached into the freezer and my hand landed on a rather leathery and warm Fudgsicle. I withdrew it to discover that I had found a wallet. I opened it up and saw the owner's address prominently displayed. His house was only half a block away from mine. Even at six I could understand that. So I toddled over and knocked on his door. The owner answered—it was a hippie dude with long hair and a beard, I remember, who stood there with his girlfriend. And as a "reward" for returning his wallet, they gave me a kitten, as their cat had recently given birth. I was so happy that I ran home with my kitten—and soon burst into tears when my mother told me we already had too many cats in the house and would have to give the kitten away. So I was soured on returning wallets from the very beginning.

You'd think that it would be common practice for people to give cash rewards for returning lost wallets—some percentage of what was in the wallet itself, most logically. You'd think. But in my long experience of returning wallets, it's happened surprisingly infrequently. Sometimes people gush with gratitude—yet no reward. And the most recent time I returned a wallet was the worst of all. I was riding a bus home from the University of California and found, under my seat, a rather thick woman's wallet. I opened it to discover that the owner—a graduate student—must have been quite well-off, because in the cash section was an eye-popping wad of $20 bills—$360 to be exact, plus several smaller bills. Wedged into a hidden area was an "emergency" $100 bill. All in all it must have totaled over $500. Never in my life had I found so much money. The other part of the wallet contained her driver's license, a great many personal effects, and no fewer than four credit cards, all platinum- or gold-colored, and all certainly not yet canceled.

Talk about tempting! But, I reasoned, I am no criminal. What am I going to do, turn to a life of crime simply because I found a wallet full of functional credit cards? I pondered keeping the cash and returning the rest of it, but that certainly would look suspicious—she'd *know* I took the cash, because if a real thief had pickpocketed her, he would have taken the cash *and* abused the credit cards before discarding the wallet. No modern thief takes just the cash and leaves the cards. So it would have had to have been the finder, me, who took the cash. Hence, I decided to give her a call and return the whole thing in toto. But her phone number was nowhere to be found. I ended up spending forty-five minutes on the Internet tracking down her phone number. I was quite sure she was freaking out with every passing minute. Oh, what joy I would bring her by returning her wallet and all of its contents! So I called her up, she answered, we arranged for her to come over to my house to pick it up, and I waited.

A full hour after the appointed time, a woman showed up at my door. She *resembled* the young woman depicted on the driver's license—yes, it was definitely she—but she had undergone a transformation in the time since the photo was taken. She had cropped her hair, dyed it blue, gotten a tattoo on her neck, and in general metamorphosed from a suburban girl into a hard-edged college radical. She said, flatly, "You called me about the wallet?" With a flourish I presented it to her, exclaiming, "You're lucky it was *me* who found it! I went to a lot of trouble to get your phone number. Here it is—it's all there. Everything!" She reached out, took it from me, said, "Okay," turned around, and got back into her car. And drove away without saying another word, or even checking the wallet, or glancing inside, or anything.

Well, *excuuuuuse* me! I had imagined tears, ecstasy, relief, rewards, rapid-fire explanations of how it was lost and found, and a reaffirmed faith in humanity. But no.

No, no, no.

I haven't found a wallet since then, but the next time I do, I will be sorely tempted to violate my own rule. So, to all you wallet losers out there: show a little gratitude to the honest scavengers who return them to you.

The situation is a little more complicated with cell phones, because it's not always obvious who owns them. At least it's not obvious to me. I am not a cell-phone user; I don't understand how they work. And they've become so sophisticated that unless you've read the manual, or are naturally adept at deciphering electronics, it's not readily apparent how to discover who the owner is. Over the last decade, I must have found at least eight cell phones, and in not a single instance was I able to return it to its rightful owner. Nor did I have any use for them. My solution in several cases was to simply place the phone back in a public place and hope the next scavenger would have the technical know-how to contact the owner. (I can be naïve at times.)

But the last one we found was a different story. Not too long ago, while out strolling, Anneli pointed to an odd object in the street. "What's that?" she asked. "Looks like one of those rubber cases for an iPhone," I said. And I was right. It *was* one of those rubber cases for an iPhone—except that when I picked it up, I discovered that *the iPhone was still inside*. Yikes. I had never owned or used an iPhone—never even touched one—but I knew they cost several hundred dollars. We brought it home and for the first few days I struggled simply to turn it on. Nothing I did seemed to have any effect. Eventually it dawned on me that its battery must have run all the way down, and it was out of juice. By sheer luck, in my box of scavenged cords and cables, I found (what I later learned was) an iPod charger cable that just happened to work with the iPhone as well. After an overnight charge and much unnecessary fiddling, I tried again, and—*shazam!*—the thing turned on. Now, if you've ever had an iPhone, you know they're more than just a phone—each one is a full-fledged mini-computer that just happens to make phone calls, if you're so inclined. I was determined, at first, to learn the identity of the owner, but I was overwhelmed by the dizzying array of options and menus. For hours I poked around, learning by trial and error, and before I could even find out the owner's name, I discovered—on his "Calendar" entries and on "sticky notes" he had left for himself—that he had permanently moved back to his home country, Brazil, the day after we had found the phone. He probably lost it while frantically preparing for the trip.

Well. Brazil. Oh gods of scavenging, do you really expect me to track down this guy's address in Brazil and FedEx him his iPhone there, at who knows what expense? Does he even care anymore? For all I know he's living on an Amazonian island in a thatch hut, surviving on açaí berries, and the last thing he wants are the trappings of civilization. Besides which, do iPhones even work in Brazil?

As I write this, the iPhone sits next to my keyboard. Yes, I decided to keep it. Am I bad? I still haven't decided whether I violated my own rule this time. Maybe through extreme effort I could have gotten the iPhone back to him, and maybe he still would have wanted it. Maybe. And maybe he would have simply said "Okay" without even offering me a berry.

7. DON'T EAT GROSS THINGS

This needs to be a rule? Even cavemen pretty much knew not to eat gross things. But culture and psychology can wield strange effects on people. And sometimes the obvious needs to be restated.

This rule is for people at the extremes: for hardcore scavengers who seem to occasionally abandon common sense when it comes to putting things in their mouths *and* for potential newcomers to the world of scavenging who are afraid that they might be pressured to eat garbage. Let's start with the second group first.

Listen carefully: If you become a scavenger, there is no compulsion to eat food out of Dumpsters. It's in there, but you don't have to take it out and you don't have to eat it. There is no scavengers' hazing ritual where you must do something revolting as a prerequisite for "joining the gang." Only a subset of scavengers ever eat any kind of scavenged food anyway. It's perfectly acceptable to embrace a scavenging identity and continue eating what you've always eaten. You can make fashion accessories out of scavenged materials or go beachcombing or prowl for bargains at thrift stores, earning your stripes as a scavenger—and still eat "normal" food bought fresh at the supermarket. It isn't necessarily an all-encompassing lifestyle.

I'm reminded of an incident long ago that had nothing to do with scavenging, really, but which illustrates the same principle. In 1978, while still a teenager, I went to a punk rock concert. But I didn't dress the part—I just wore my same old dorky 1978 clothes. Awareness of the new punk fashions had just reached our town, and as I entered the concert, I saw many other kids—including kids I knew who normally sported bell-bottoms and long hair—dressed up in their best approximation of this new style. Soon after entering I was challenged by some jerk with a mohawk who said, "What are you doing here? You aren't a punk!" Of course, he hadn't been a punk either until a few weeks earlier. But you know how new converts are. I answered, "I'm not claiming to be a punk. I just like the music." He snorted in derision, but the confrontation stayed with me. Because over the following few years, kids across America declared their fidelity to this or that music style by wearing the appropriate "fashion uniform." But I never did. Even though I went to punk rock shows and followed the bands' careers like many other people of my generation, I never adopted the punk "lifestyle," nor did I ever look punk or anything even close.

And the same holds true for modern-day scavengers. Even if you like some aspect of scavenging, you don't need to "look like a scavenger," and you certainly don't need to *eat* like a scavenger, either.

At the other end of the scale are those for whom the scavenging identity is everything. You know who you are. And to such people it becomes almost a challenge to see if an entire diet can be composed of scavenged food. If food was somehow obtained legitimately, these folks reject it as ideologically impure. Politically and ecologically, they're purists. And—some would say ironically—they manifest their purism by Dumpster diving for food. Every day, they test the limits of what might be edible. How bruised or fuzzy is the fruit? How far past its expiration date is the bacon?

Our advice is: Stop for a moment and think about what you're doing. No one is going to condemn you for not being scavengeologically pure. You don't need to prove yourself. The last thing you want is to end up in the hospital with salmonella.

8. DON'T BRAG OR BROWBEAT OTHERS; SCAVENGING IS NOT FOR EVERYBODY

Even if you've grown proud of your scavenger lifestyle or hobby, try to resist becoming a Scavenging Snob. It's not a good way to win converts.

As a point of comparison, acquaintances who learn that I'm a vegetarian sometimes ask, if we're at a picnic or a barbecue, "You don't mind if I eat meat, do you?" I always find this an astonishing question. "Of course not," I tell them. "Eat whatever you want. I merely decide what *I* eat; I don't dictate what other people eat." Then they end up being amazed at my laissez-faire attitude; they tell me that other vegetarians they've encountered *do* in fact try to pressure everyone around them into not eating meat. Or, even more annoyingly, act like they can't even be around the smell of meat and pout by refusing to eat at all unless they're in a completely meatfree environment. And some even go so far as to lecture the carnivores around them on the evils of the meat industry.

This kind of holier-than-thou attitude usually ends up backfiring: if you berate or browbeat people over something, often their urge is to do the exact opposite of what you had hoped—just to show you what a pain in the butt you're being.

So if someone shows off a new painting she bought at an art

gallery for $2,000, never try to humiliate her by bragging that *you* got a wild example of outsider art at a thrift store for a mere fifty cents. Instead, show your appreciation of the expensive art, and later, *if the topic comes up,* you can mention in a noncompetitive way that you collect paint-by-number clown portraits from the 1970s. But claiming that your clowns are inherently superior to someone else's Picassos will only earn you enemies.

Remember that scavenging is not for everybody. And it *can't* be for everybody, or we'd all be squabbling over the same limited secondhand resources. If you want to gently lead others into a scavenging mindset, lead by example—not by bullying or braggadocio.

9. DON'T POACH THINGS FROM OTHER SCAVENGERS

This is actually a corollary of the first commandment. Once another scavenger has claimed something, it becomes his or her possession; if you poach it, then you are in essence stealing. If you are at a garage sale at the end of the day and the seller has announced that everything left is free or almost free, and several scavengers are scrambling around making caches of stuff to keep, don't snag something from another scavenger's cache when his or her back is turned. And if, in another circumstance, you see something that has been put out on the street and labeled for a nonprofit or charity to pick up, just leave it there, no matter how tempting it might be.

The most common form that poaching takes among impoverished scavengers is to abscond with the bottles, cans, and newspapers that homeowners leave for the municipal recycling service to pick up. There is an ongoing debate as to whether or not this is illegal, since by putting it out on the street the homeowner has forfeited ownership of the material; yet the new owner has not yet taken possession. Either way, recycling poachers often draw complaints because they sometimes leave a big mess when they're done, and usually make an even bigger racket at five in the morning, dumping bottles and cans into a shopping cart or the back of a truck. I realize that to such people economic necessity takes precedence over courtesy, but I think it's important to say that early-morning recyclables poaching is against scavenger ethics, even if the prohibition isn't likely to be heeded.

10. DO NOT SCAM

In a sense, this too is actually part of Rule 1, because scamming is a form of stealing, whether the victim being scammed into giving away goods or money under false pretenses is a charity, a nonprofit, a religious or academic institution, a private business, an individual, or the government.

Lying about your circumstances in order to extract something from others is deceptive, manipulative, and totally immoral. It's not simply a lie, which in any case is ethically iffy enough. It's a lie that causes harm, in that it deprives the giver of goods or capital, impoverishing the giver in principle, even if the giver is rich and generous. It also harms other potential recipients *who actually deserve the largesse.* Their very survival might depend on whatever money, materials, or other benefits the giver has to give. If by trickery a scammer has gotten the money, materials, or other benefits for himself or herself, then that portion cannot be given to those who are genuinely needy.

That's theft.

Lying about your circumstances, claiming to be poor when you're not (or at least poorer than you actually are), claiming to be unemployed when you're not, claiming to be disabled when you're not, claiming to support more dependents than you're supporting, claiming to live somewhere where you don't actually live—these are classic and all-too-common scams perpetrated with the aim of getting free stuff. And they're all too often successful, resulting in massive quantities doled out in benefits, scholarships, handouts, free food, free housing, free medical care, and aid programs of every stripe. Getting such aid because you're destitute without it is one thing. Lying to get it is larcenous greed.

Oh, and lying to the U.S. government is a federal crime.

11. DON'T BE A MOOCHER

Scavenging is *supposed* to be about serendipity: finding things that Lady Luck puts in your path. And sure, you can guide yourself through life in such a way that increases your chances of not-so-randomly acquiring things for free. But one must become very careful not to cross the line into moocherdom. Because nobody likes a mooch.

You know you've become a moocher when you consciously target specific individuals to be the sources of your "scavenged" acquisitions. You'll hang around kindhearted or well-off suckers and act needy or desperate. And whenever they offer you something, you *always* take them up on it. And then you just keep coming back for more.

That's not being a scavenger—that's being a parasite. And as mentioned in Chapter 2, the only creatures with a worse reputation than scavengers are parasites.

The same principle holds true at parties or weddings or buffet luncheons. It's fine to browse the food table, as everybody is expected to, scavenging a free meal. It's quite another to park yourself at the buffet and scarf down all the prawns, especially when there is a limited amount of each dish. If you're going to party-crash just for the scavenging thrill of it (and you shouldn't, because that's trespassing), at least be discreet.

Some people develop an entire lifestyle based on mooching, and it can get ugly. And to the extent that such people are identified as scavengers, they give us all a bad name. So for the sake of your own dignity, don't become an interpersonal parasite. If you simply can't help being a moocher, please don't use the scavenging movement as a cover for your behavior.

12. DON'T BRING SHAME ONTO SCAVENGERS AND SCAVENGING

This is not really a separate rule unto itself. Rather, it's a summation of all the rules above. If you're going to follow only one scavenging principle, let it be this one: *Act in a way that brings credit to scavengers as a group.* Always keep in mind the notion that, if you identify as a scavenger, when you embarrass yourself, you're embarrassing all of us.

HERE'S A STAND-ALONE LIST of Scavenging Dos and Don'ts—or to be more grandiose, Scavenging Commandments:

Obey the law.
Don't be aggressive or abusive.
Always clean up after yourself.

Don't harm plants, animals, or people.

Learn from your finds.

Don't live like a slob.

Appreciate the small things.

Don't endanger your health.

Be someone that others would want to emulate.

Don't become a creepy eccentric.

Help the planet.

Don't be a parasite.

Be modest.

Be courteous.

Don't steal.

EPILOGUE

I was Lord of the whole Mannor; or if I pleas'd, I might call my self King, or Emperor over the whole Country which I had Possession of. There were no Rivals. I had no Competitor, none to dispute Sovereignty or Command with me. . . . I had Grapes enough to have made Wine, or to have cur'd into Raisins, to have loaded that Fleet, when they had been built. But all I could make use of, was, All that was valuable. I had enough to eat, and to supply my Wants, and, what was all the rest to me? . . . In a Word, The Nature and Experience of Things dictated to me upon just Reflection, That all the good Things of this World, are no farther good to us, than they are for our Use; and that whatever we may heap up indeed to give others, we enjoy just as much as we can use, and no more. The most covetous griping Miser in the World would have been cur'd of the Vice of Covetousness, if he had been in my Case; for I possess'd infinitely more than I knew what to do with. I had no room for Desire, except it was of Things which I had not, and they were but Trifles, though indeed of great Use to me. . . . All our Discontents about what we want, appear'd to me, to spring from the Want of Thankfulness for what we have.

—DANIEL DEFOE, *Robinson Crusoe*

WE FOUND A DIAMOND RING.

We have both always dreamed of finding diamond rings: literally dreamed, waking with fingers flexed. The fact that one of us never wears jewelry and the other already wears a diamond engagement ring inherited from a grandmother is irrelevant.

Since childhood, we have dreamed of finding diamond rings. It is a childish dream, totally juvenile, like something in a fairy tale. Of all the things a scavenger could wish for, all the miraculous helpful things—a formula for curing AIDS, the Amber Room, a map pinpointing the Roanoke Colony, Atlantis, the real Grail. But no. For us: the ring. We had found other types of rings, enough to fill two jars. Carnelian, garnet, plain silver, plain gold, plain copper, turquoise, jet, jade, pearl. But never diamond. We met *other* scavengers who'd found them. Of course, it meant hardly anything to them. They'd sold the rings or given them to women who had broken up with them and taken the rings when they went. *Of course.*

So then we found one!

We were walking down a residential street we seldom take. It is lined with fanciful faux chalets and haciendas. Crossing a street named for a philosopher, we saw three boxes lined up on the curb. A woman with a dog bent over one. We tensed up. Rivalry. *She got there first.*

But she stood and walked off, bearing a single empty picture frame. We rushed across the street and reached the boxes. What had she left behind? We pulled things out and began dropping them into our backpacks. Oven mitts. A salad spinner. Crocheted scarves. And then: a little wooden box with a flower painted on it. *Huh, what's in here?*

Diamond ring.

It was a solitaire, worn long and hard, its gold rim paper-thin. Under that liquid sky it slipped right on. A perfect fit.

What do you do when dreams come true? Spread your arms wide and whirl?

Not us. We felt suffused with light. Not that the ring looked valuable. Stone bright but the size of a mustard seed. Rim thin. Yet it had come to us. Right there, right then.

This was the moment we'd been waiting for.

We needed nothing but to know this.

Who would give away a diamond ring? The furious, the airheaded, the spurned? The boxes stood pert on the curb, like hundreds more that we had seen all over town before. These three did not say FREE, but some FREE boxes don't.

An angry ex? *This is how much I care about you, bastard.* A rebellious teen? *Ha ha, Mom, I threw out your heirloom.* Strange stuff gets discarded all the time. Valuable stuff. Once we were walking down another street where a woman was emptying the contents of her house into a Dumpster. Helter-skelter, like. Armloads of power tools, armloads of folded sheets, armloads of suits. We watched a fur coat and a mah-jongg set go in. She said her husband had died suddenly two weeks before. *I can't stand to see our stuff anymore.* The house was up for sale. *I'll make a clean break.*

She invited us to climb inside. *Take what you want.* That day we wound up with a closetful of clothes, a box of nautical souvenirs—boat whistles, flags, a little wooden fisherman—and pocketfuls of change. She was throwing away his change. She would not take it back.

So, honestly, giving away a diamond ring—why not?

It felt like an emblem of membership. This simple ring without flourishes was a milestone. *Hark, you have arrived.*

The stone was not just small but flawed. But it was found and it was free. Our miracle. What might it portend? We scared ourselves, pondering whether, when ultimate dreams come true, the dreamers promptly die.

A week later, we walked down the same street again. Really, we almost never walk there. It was happenstance. We almost *never*—

Pinned to telephone poles along the street were signs. "PLEASE HELP! THE BOXES THAT WERE HERE ON FRIDAY 5/16 WERE NOT MEANT TO BE FREE!!!!!! WE WERE MOVING AND THE MOVERS LEFT THEM BEHIND. THE CONTENTS HAD SENTIMENTAL VALUE ESPE-CIALLY MY MOTHER'S RING. REWARD." And then a phone number.

What do we do when dreams implode? We call.

When we handed it back, she wept. We would not take the whole reward but settled for a third of it. To us, twenty bucks is a lot. She was young and sweet, and her boyfriend, looking so relieved behind her, gave a sideways grin and made flamboyant praying hands.

THE NEXT ONE will be platinum.

NOTES

Chapter 3 THE OLDEST PROFESSION

page 59 In his 1935 novel *Untouchable*: Mulk Raj Anand, *Untouchable* (New York: Penguin, 1941).

page 68 In his memoir *The Old Home Town*: Izhak Ze'ev Jonis, *The Old Home Town*, part of the Mlawa Remembrance Initiative; http://www.zchor.org/MLAW7.HTM.

page 69 In *How the Other Half Lives*: Jacob A. Riis, *How the Other Half Lives* (New York: Charles Scribner's Sons, 1890).

page 71 Typical was a new law: "With Carts in Tow, Street Scavengers Brace for Crackdown," Agence France-Presse, March 2, 2008.

page 73 "The fireplace is built of stones and mud": Louise Amelia Knapp Smith Clappe, *The Shirley Letters* (Berkeley, CA: Heyday Books, 1998).

page 76 A resident of Pittsburgh: S. Lee Kann, *Show Places and Know Places in Pittsburgh* (Pittsburgh: Lee-Art, 1932).

Chapter 4 SCAVENOMICS

page 96 Social historian Susan Strasser examines the mostly forgotten story: Susan Strasser, *Waste and Want: A Social History of Trash* (New York: Henry Holt, 2001).

page 105 As Carl Zimring details in his history of scrap dealers: Carl A. Zimring, *Cash for Your Trash: Scrap Recycling in America* (Piscataway, NJ: Rutgers University Press, 2005).

Chapter 5 **FOUND STYLE**

page 115 "Japhy's clothes were all old hand-me-downs": Jack Kerouac, *The Dharma Bums* (New York: Penguin, 2000).

page 119 In an interview about hippie fashion: Angela Cooke, "A Bit Tight Around the Hippies," *The Sunday Mirror,* September 14, 2008.

page 121 Their plan was to excite the masses: The Digger Papers, http://www.diggers.org/digpaps68/dp_memo.html.

page 122 The troupe's founder, R. G. Davis, defines his inspiration: Dominic Cavallo, *It's Free Because It's Yours* (New York: St. Martin's Press, 1999).

page 123 Reflecting on the New York store: Marty Jezer, *Abbie Hoffman, American Rebel* (Piscataway, NJ: Rutgers University Press, 1993).

page 124 "In perhaps the most pointless robbery": Charles Perry, *The Haight-Ashbury: A History* (New York: Random House, 1984).

page 125 Janis Joplin, observed one journalist: Peter Reilly, "The Double-Edged Soul of Janis Joplin," *Stereo Review*, January 1, 1970.

page 125 In 1967, at the murderous apex of China's Cultural Revolution: James F. Coyne, "The Follies That Come with Spring," *Time*, March 24, 1967.

page 125 One such seeker was Jane Ormsby-Gore: Series of interviews conducted by the Victoria & Albert Museum, http://www.vam.ac.uk/collections/fashion/features/1960s/interviews.

page 131 "I sold the ruins of pop culture": Malcolm McLaren, "Dirty Pretty Things," *Guardian*, May 28, 2004.

page 132 "That black school blazer I renovated late last night": Paul Marko, *The Roxy London WC2: A Punk History* (London: Punk 77, 2007).

page 135 When Nirvana front man Kurt Cobain committed suicide: Timothy Egan, "Kurt Cobain, Hesitant Poet of 'Grunge Rock,' Dead at 27," *New York Times*, April 9, 1994.

page 138 The sexually inquisitive young heroine: Haruki Murakami, *Sputnik Sweetheart* (New York: Vintage, 2002).

page 141 There they are resold again and again: Michael Durham, "Clothes Line," *Guardian*, February 25, 2004.

page 141 Anthropologist and material-culture expert Karen Tranberg Hansen: Luz Claudio, "Waste Couture," *Environmental Health Perspectives*, September 2007.

page 142 "These clothes make people's dreams come true": Davan Maharaj, "For Sale, Cheap—Dead White Men's Clothing," *Los Angeles Times*, July 14, 2004.

page 146 "Lindsay Lohan sizzles in racy photo shoot": Tammy Lovell, *Daily Mail*, June 9, 2008.

page 146 In March 2007, under the headline: "Thrift Like a Celebrity," *Glamour*, March 14, 2007.

page 146 Interviewed during Paris fashion week: "Dame Helen: I Still Love a Bargain," *Daily Express*, July 3, 2008.

Chapter 6 FINDING YOURSELF

page 161 One such test, commissioned in 2005: Elizabeth Olson, "The Growing Cachet of the Store Brand," *New York Times*, November 27, 2005.

page 172 Founded by a group of artists: The Fallen Fruit Manifesto, http://www.fallenfruit.org.

page 184 In Alexandre Dumas's *The Count of Monte Cristo*: Alexandre Dumas, *The Count of Monte Cristo* (New York: Penguin, 2003).

Chapter 8 THE ACCIDENTAL TAOIST

page 216 In the story, a poor Hawaiian buys: Robert Louis Stevenson, *Travels in Hawaii* (Honolulu: University of Hawaii Press, 1991).

page 218 In Navajo tradition, for instance, corpses are washed: Gladys A. Reichard, *The Social Life of the Navajo Indians with Some Attention to Minor Ceremonies* (Whitefish, MT: Kessinger, 2006).

page 228 "Almost all of the creatures on the unclean list are scavengers": David L. Meinz, *Eating by the Book: What the Bible Says About Food, Fat,*

Fitness and Faith (Washington, DC: National Nutrition Services, 1999).

page 234 The all-time classic scavenging novel: Daniel Defoe, *Robinson Crusoe* (New York: Modern Library, 2001).

page 236 This Sufi tale, translated: Idries Shah, *Tales of the Dervishes* (New York: Penguin, 2003).

page 240 Its qualities, its imponderable order-within-apparent-chaos: Lao Tzu and Stephen Mitchell, *Tao Te Ching* (New York: Harper Perennial, 2006); and an e-book version by Ron Hogan, http://www.beatrice.com/TAO.html.

INDEX